LEAN AND GREEN

DIET COOKBOOK

3 Books in 1

The Master Guide to Lose Weight in Critical Points, Increase Energy with Healthy, Super Fast and Enjoyable Recipes and a Weight Maintenance Program with Easy Shopping Lists.

Table Of Contents

LEAN AND GREEN DIET

LEAN AND GREEN DIET FOR WEIGHT LOSS

LEAN AND GREEN COOKBOOK 2021

LEAN AND GREEN DIET

A Complete Guide With A 21-Day Plan To Lose Pounds In A Simple, Fast And Definitive Way Without Counting Calories, Includes A Weight Maintenance Program With Easy Shopping Lists

Introduction

Lean and Green diet is a popular meal replacement program that participants have confirmed

is very useful in rapid weight loss. The diet is observed by combining "Fuelings" (such as bars, shakes, and many other pre-packaged foods) with a six-small-meals-per-day principle to help people lose weight without going through strenuous exercises but consuming calories in a minimal amount throughout the day.

There is also provision for a health coach that the consumer can relate with, and he or she will guide the consumer while taking the diet program and will give support, motivation, and encouragement.

Several "Lean and Green" recipes you will be eating while taking the program are also provided, and with this, you can enjoy the best of this diet program.

Lean and Green diet enhances weight loss through branded products known as "Fuelings" while the homemade entrées are referred to as the "Lean and Green" meals. The Fuelings are made up of over 60 items, specifically low in carbs (carbohydrates) but high in probiotic cultures and protein. The fuelings ultimately contain friendly bacteria that can help boost gut health. They include cookies, bars, puddings, shakes, soups, cereals, and pasta.

Looking at the listed foods, you might think they are relatively high in carbs, which is understandable, but the Fuelings are composed so that they are lower in sugar and carbs than the traditional versions of similar foods. The company does this by using small-portion sizes and sugar substitutes. Many of the Fuelings are packed with soy protein isolate and whey protein powder in furtherance. Those who are interested in the Lean and Green diet plan but are not interested in cooking or have no chance for it are provided with pre-made, low-carb meals. These meals are referred to as "Flavors of Home," and they can sufficiently replace the Lean and Green Meals.

The company explicitly states that by working with its team of coaches and following the Lean and Green diet as required, you will achieve a "lifelong transformation, one healthy habit at a time."

Therefore, to record success with this diet plan, you have to stick to the Fuelings supplemented by veggie, meat, and healthy fat entrée daily; you will be full and nourished. Although you will be consuming low calories, you will not be losing a lot of muscle since you will be feeding on lots of fiber, protein, and other vital nutrients. Your calories as an adult will not exceed 800–1,000. You can lose 12 pounds in 12 weeks if you follow the 5&1 Optimal Weight Plan option.

Since you will curb your carb intake while on this diet plan, you will naturally shed fat because the carb is the primary source of energy, therefore, if it is not readily available, the body finds a fat alternative, which implies that the body will have to break down your fats for energy and keep burning fat.

Finally, with this book, you will determine if the Lean and Green diet program is a weight loss program convenient for you before you get started.

"I'm on a diet. I can't come for the weekend!" Punctually said Martha, a friend I have known since adolescence. She was always struggling with weight; she never saw herself right, and when we went out with the others, she had constant difficulties in choosing fashionable clothes like all of us. In reality, he didn't have that many kg in excess... maybe 5–6...? But this caused her low self-esteem and insecurity in any social context. After 27 years of diets, she got married and had a beautiful baby. Martha, during pregnancy, gained 30 kilograms! So that suffering resurfaces for her appearance, for the joint pains that lead her not to sleep at night, lethargy, and that sense of discomfort with her husband who saw her only with those XXL clothes. She was tired of diets that started on Monday and stopped for the weekend. She needed a fast, definitive, serious path, but above all, a support that would help her manage meals because now, with a family, she couldn't stop cooking and isolate herself.

So she knew the Lean and Green Diet, a low-carb path with a high-protein content, and is immediately struck because it was based on a choice of over 60 healthy and fast solutions, including shakes, bars, soups, biscuits, salty snacks ... high content protein, with probiotics and prebiotics to promote correct absorption of nutrients and good digestion. In this way, she no longer had to waste time and money in supermarkets, looking for refined and unavailable ingredients!! She could choose between 3 different routes that would bring her to a healthy weight. Martha chose the strongest and fastest 5&1, moving on to 4&2&1 and then to 3&3. It is a path that is not based only on substitute meals but also on cooked meals, precisely to not become slaves to a product and learn to eat while losing weight healthily, not affecting lean mass. After a short time, her appearance began to change, not only for the loss of weight and size, but for that radiant light on her face, different energy, and for the first time I saw her sitting at the table serene, without having to give up her social life. This book is for all those women who often step aside, at the expense of their happiness, but who deserve a new chance.

Martha finally found her solution with the Lean and Green diet, eliminating those 30 kgs in a few months and entering the size 40 she had always sought. To date, after two years, it has never started again, dispelling the myth that by following low-calorie routes, one gains weight quickly. First of all, because with this diet you eat 6 times a day and the kg you recover is determined exclusively by the incorrect lifestyle, you are applying at that moment and not by the previous one. This book also serves as mental support on approaching a definitive path of transformation and is perhaps my favorite part because it is essential to keep in mind why you started and where you want to go. I believe that each of us deserves to feel better, feel full of energy, and not underestimate ourselves as a woman!!

And since we women like to share our secrets, here you can find many: on how not to finally give up on social life, how to organize yourself with meals, how to meet the needs of the whole family, how to find yourself without guilt and many healthy, practical and tasty recipes that will lead you to be satisfied even in the kitchen, regaining your physical shape, and without having to count calories anymore! You will have a list of foods to prefer and avoid that you can always carry with you and some practical tricks on smart shopping! We will start with the first action: cleaning the kitchen pantries of all those pre-packaged foods, which intoxicate us, make room for healthy foods, and combine them in a conscious, stimulating, and fun way! And then, let's face it: the healthier you eat, the more your body will ask for healthy things! Enjoy this book and your wellness journey with the Lean and Green diet!

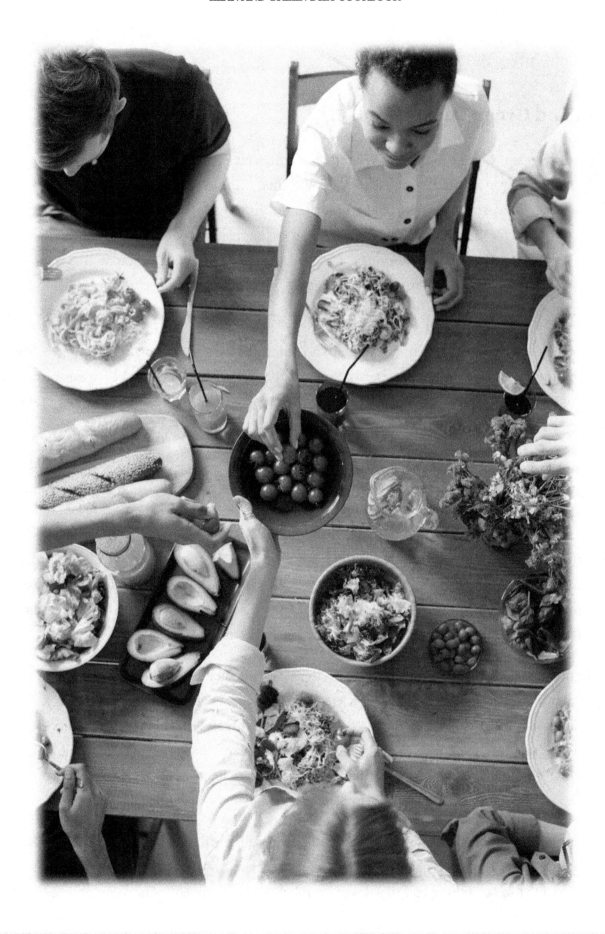

Lean and Green Diet's Mindset

As you know, you will not lose weight overnight, so it's good to keep a mindset that every day counts even if you can't see it on the scale. Just think of it as one big step closer, even if it feels like a small step. I would advise you not to weigh yourself every day as this may put you off, and any progress might seem like it's happening too slow. Stick to once a week at the same time in the mornings. If you do weigh yourself at different times, do not be alarmed if you seem to put on weight, as it can and will fluctuate during the day and throughout the week. This is because of the things you consume and how your body handles them.

You can also look at it as a game or challenge to become fun rather than something you hate. The best way to do this is to find another person to share your progress with. This can be friends or family or even people you don't know and sometimes a group. Because you have the same goals as other people out there, you may even make some new friends.

You can make certain meals feel like a treat even though they are nowhere near as bad as some of your usual eating habits, but you can still fill that desire. Moderation and better choices come into play here, so don't order the burger and fries. Have a chicken salad instead.

Every time you look in the fridge and spot something you really shouldn't be eating, think of that food in the future and not the present. It may taste nice when you eat it, but you will feel guilty afterward, and a few days after that, the scale may not show the progress you wanted it to show, so just think ahead of time before making any decision when making food choices.

People may make fun of you for choosing to exercise and diet. They may not believe in you for whatever reason. This may be because they could not imagine themselves changing their lifestyle in such a way, so in their eyes, you must also fail at it. Shrug it off and continue as usual, and you will be the one laughing when you reach your goals. It's not an issue what other people think as it's your actions that dictate your outcome. To achieve this, you need to let go of all your fears that could make it harder for you and concentrate on the result.

Sometimes when you are doing well, you may treat yourself a little too much, and then it backfires, and you end up doing more damage to your progress than you could have imagined. Instead of treating yourself to something bad to eat, you could challenge yourself to have something healthy in place of that treat and then feel twice as good later. Self-satisfaction is the biggest reward. Remember, it's still excellent to treat yourself every now and again to avoid binging. Have a cheat meal or a cheat day but fit it into your daily calorie limit.

Sticking to Good Habits

Most people want to be the best person they can be. They want to live healthy, well-rounded lives that satisfy them. They usually all know what they SHOULD be doing on a day-to-day basis to achieve this life they desire. So why is it so hard to stick to good habits? Why do we get motivated for short periods only to fall back into bad habits a short time later?

Have you ever resolved to add a healthy habit to your life? Lose 20 pounds? Eat healthier? Increase the amount of weight you can lift? Chances are, if you are like most, you started those practices with the best intentions, only to get sidetracked somewhere along the way, and they never became habits. Why does that happen so consistently to so many of us? The answer is that we try to make changes in the wrong way. In attempting to change the wrong way, there is little possibility for something to become a lasting change. This book will show you a better strategy to finally make long term changes in your life successfully.

Do's & Don'ts of the Lean and Green Diet

The Lean and Green diet plan has some guidelines—especially in food consumption—that must be adhered to if you wish to record a diet plan successfully.

Recommended Foods to Eat

The foods you are liable to eat while on the 5&1 plan are the 5 Lean and Green Fuelings and 1 Lean and Green meal dail

The meals consist mainly of healthy fats, lean protein, and low-carb vegetables, and there is a recommendation for only two servings of fatty fish every week. Some beverages and low-carb condiments are also allowed in small proportions.

The Foods that Are allowed for the Lean and Green Meals

- **Fish and Shellfish:** Trout, tuna, halibut, salmon, crab, scallops, lobster, and shrimp

- **Meat:** Lean beef, lamb, chicken, game meats, turkey, tenderloin or pork chop, and ground meat (must be 85% lean at least)
- **Vegetable Oils:** Walnut, flaxseed, olive oil, and canola
- **Eggs:** Whole Eggs, egg beaters, and egg whites
- **Additional Healthy Fats:** Reduced-fat margarine, walnuts, pistachios, almonds, avocado, olives, and low carb salad dressings
- **Soy Products:** Tofu
- **Sugar-free Beverages:** Unsweetened almond milk, coffee, tea, and water
- **Sugar-free Snacks:** Gelatin, mints, popsicles, and gum
- **Low-Carb Vegetables:** Celery, mushrooms, cauliflower, zucchini, peppers, jicama, spinach, cucumbers, cabbage, eggplant, broccoli, spaghetti squash, and collard greens
- **Seasonings and Condiments:** Lemon juice, yellow mustard, salsa, zero-calorie sweeteners, barbecue sauce, cocktail sauce, dried herbs, salt, spices, lime juice, soy sauce, sugar-free syrup, and ½ teaspoons only of ketchup

Summary: The Lean and Green 5&1 plan's homemade meals consist mainly of low-carb veggies, lean proteins, and a few healthy fats. It allows only low-carb beverages like unsweetened almond milk, water, tea, and coffee.

Foods That Are Not Allowed

Apart from the carbs contained in the pre-packaged Lean and Green fuelings, most carb-containing beverages and foods are not allowed while you are on the 5&1 plan. Some fats are also banned as well as all fried foods.

Below are the foods you must avoid, except if they are included in your Fuelings:

- **Refined Grains:** Pasta, pancakes, crackers, cookies, pastries, white bread, biscuits, flour tortillas, white rice, and cakes
- **Fried Foods:** Fish, vegetables, shellfish, meats, and sweets like pastries
- **Whole Fat Dairy:** Cheese, milk, and yogurt
- **Certain Fats:** Coconut oil, butter, and solid shortening

- **Sugar-Sweetened Beverages:** fruit juice, soda, energy drinks, sports drinks, and sweet tea
- **Alcohol:** All varieties

The foods below are banned while on the 5&1 plan but are added to the 6-week transition phase and with no restriction during the 3&3 plan:

- **Fruits:** All fresh fruits
- **Whole Grains:** High-fibre breakfast cereal, whole grain bread, whole-wheat pasta, and brown rice
- **Starch Vegetables:** Corn, white potatoes, sweet potatoes, and peas
- **Low-Fat or Fat-Free Dairy:** Milk, yogurt, and cheese
- **Legumes:** Beans, peas, lentils, and soybeans

Note that during the 6-week transition phase, and while on the 3&3 plan, you are advised to eat more berries if you must take fruits as they contain lower carbs.

Fundamentals of Lean and Green Diet

Lean and Green is a fast weight reduction or maintenance method that prescribes a combination of bought, refined foods labeled "Fueling" and "Lean and Green" home-made meals. There's no carbohydrates or calories counting. Instead, as part of six-or-so small meals every day, members apply water to a powdered meal or unwrap a cookie.

The purpose of introducing Fuelings is to curb the cravings and a nutritiously balanced meal to keep the dieter satiated.

Based on the requirements of a person, there are three different low-calorie strategies to choose from.

1. The 5&1 plan requires 5 Lean and Green Fuelings and 1 Lean and Green meal, and it consists of vegetables and proteins (for example, broccoli and chicken), which are included in the 5&1 Program.
2. The 4&2&1 strategy requires 4 Fuelings, 2 Lean and Green meals, and 1 light snack (like a slice of fruit) for a bit more variety.

3. The 3&3 package, which involves 3 Fuelings and 3 Lean and Green products, for those participating in weight management.

Lean and Green also presents trainers with instructions to help you develop their "Habits of Health." The strategy also advises performing approximately 30 minutes of exercise with mild intensity every day and consuming more than 64 ounces of water daily.

This Lean and Green diet is meant to help individuals reduce weight and obesity by portion-controlled snacks and meals by lowering carbohydrates and calories.

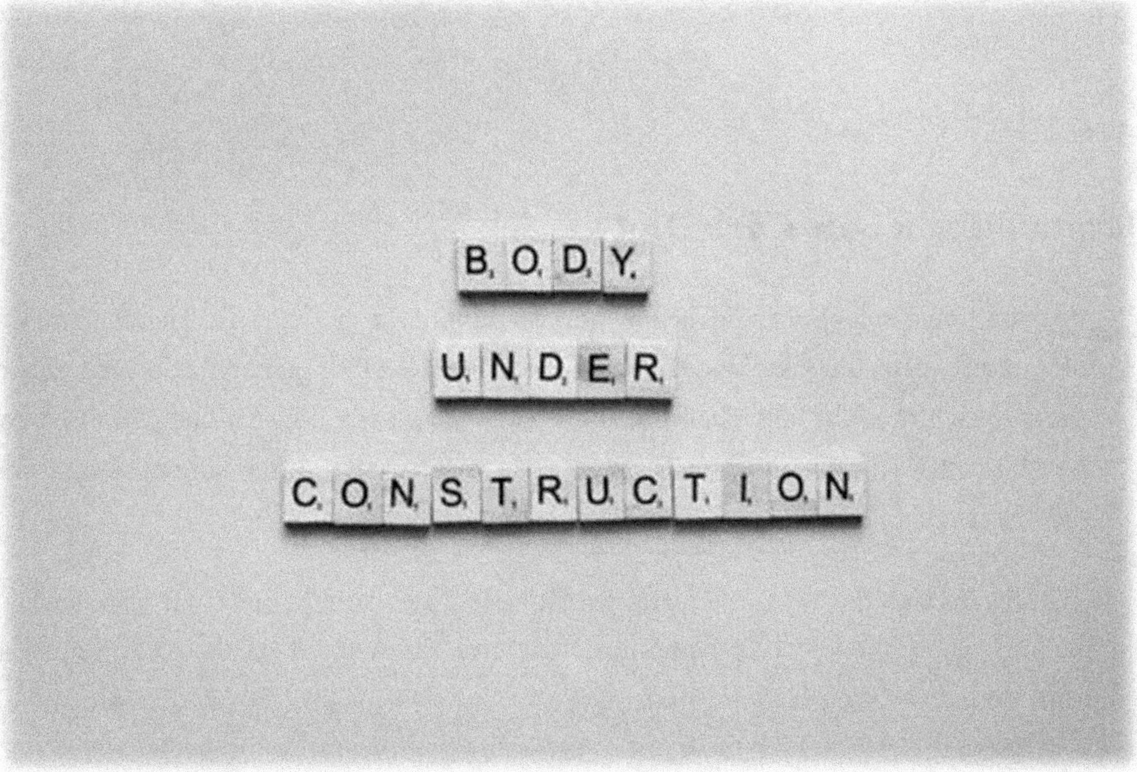
BODY
UNDER
CONSTRUCTION

LOW CARB

Understanding a Low-Carb Diet

The definition of a low-carb diet is one that has minimal carbohydrates. There are many types of low-carb diets, but the ones that proved to be beneficial to managing diabetes substituted the carbs with healthy fats. That way, it becomes a low-carb, high-fat diet. If you are going to cut the carbs, you need to provide your body with an alternative energy source, which is healthy fats in this case.

That means significantly minimizing or cutting out high-starch foods and carbs such as rice, pasta, processed sugary foods, foods containing flour, like white bread, while loading up your diet with high-fiber and low-glycemic-index foods such as vegetables, healthy fats, and proteins to a lesser extent.

Managing your weight with a low-carb diet is a healthy way to lose weight and promote your overall health. It converts your body from being a sugar-burning machine into a fat-burning machine. However, note that there is a transition period of about 7 to 14 days before your body wholly and successfully switches from burning sugars to burning fats. During this transition period, your body will suffer from mild changes due to carbs deprivation (remember, it still depends on carbs during the transition period).

Problems with a Low-Carb Diet

You will also face initial fatigue from the shift in your diet and lower your glucose intake. If you have type 1 diabetes, you need to be very careful about making dietary habit changes. This requires modification of your insulin dose, so you need to consult your doctor before making any diet changes. The fewer carbohydrates you ingest, the less insulin you will need, and therefore, you will not need the same amount of insulin dose you used to take when you were having a regular or high-carb diet.

As your body transitions from a high-carb state to a low-carb state, you will face some problems, but this should not discourage you. Here is a list of issues that you may face in the short transition period when you initially start a low-carb diet:

You may start to feel lightheaded or dizzy, get headaches or feel fatigued, but this will quickly go away within a few days as your body starts to adapt to using fats for energy instead of sugars. If this problem persists or affects your normal daily functions, stop the low-carb diet immediately, and consult your doctor.

You may find yourself having problems with retaining water, as the carbohydrates help in water retention. When you decrease your carb intake, you will start to shed more water than your body typically loses. Loss of water is often accompanied by loss of salt; this may lead you to feel cramps or experience rapid heartbeats. You may also feel your pressure drop due to the loss of water. You can compensate by drinking lots of water and adding minerals to it. These changes are only temporary and should subside after some time; however, if you remain tired, dizzy, or sleepy, consult your doctor immediately.

Aren't Fats Unhealthy?

We mentioned that it is important to include fat in the replacement of the decreased carb intake. This raises the question, "aren't fats unhealthy?" It is a misconception to assume that fats are unhealthy. They are an essential component in our body. Your body needs fats to synthesize many hormones—and this goes into the composition of our cell membrane. Fats are also heat-insulators, preserving your body's heat. They also lie around your vital organs, such as the kidney, protecting it from trauma. A moderate amount of fat is necessary for a healthy body. However, the problem with fats occurs when they exceed the normal range.

There are healthy fats and unhealthy fats. The same goes for cholesterol. There is good cholesterol and bad cholesterol. Fish, olive oil and eggs, etc., contain natural fats. However, synthetic hydrogenated fats are considered an unhealthy type.

Good cholesterol is associated with HDL (high-density lipoprotein), which is a healthy and desirable type of cholesterol, as it helps lower your lipids and improve your lipid profile. This contrasts with LDL (low-density lipoprotein), which has undesirable health effects on your body. Therefore, it is essential to distinguish between the different types of fats to know what foods to opt for and what foods to avoid. Examples of healthy fats include monounsaturated fats and polyunsaturated fats.

Examples of Monounsaturated Fats

- Avocados, olives, peanut butter, oils like sesame oil, peanut oil, canola oil, and olive oil

- Nuts like peanuts, almonds, hazelnuts, pecans, and cashews

Examples of Polyunsaturated Fats

- Sunflower seeds, sesame seeds, and pumpkin seeds

- Nuts like walnuts

- Fatty fish like salmon, tuna, mackerel, sardines, and fish oil

- Plant oils like soya bean and safflower oil

- Tofu and soya milk

Examples of unhealthy fats include trans fats and saturated fats.

Examples of Trans Fats

- All the commercially-baked cookies, doughnuts, pastries, muffins, pizza dough, etc.

- Packaged snacks such as microwave popcorn, chips, or crackers

- Hydrogenated margarine

- Fried food such as fried chicken, chicken nuggets, breaded fish, and French fries

- Food that contains hydrogenated vegetable oils

Examples of Saturated Fats

- Chicken skin

- Hydrogenated butter

- Ice cream

- Fatty meat

General Habits to Decrease Your Carb Intake

There are many ways to decrease your carb intake. Everything lies in the small habits, especially your shopping habits, as that is where it all begins. When you are shopping, avoid items like bakeries in general and pastries full of carbs. Instead, load up your shopping cart with vegetables. Did you know that you can have 20 grams of carbs by either a plateful of assorted vegetables or a slice of bread? Guess which one makes you feel fuller and which one is healthier?

Start substituting main course items with healthy alternatives. For example, you can replace rice with cauliflower by grinding it in a blender to make cauliflower rice. It is almost the same and is much healthier.

You can also replace the pastries in your shopping cart with healthy alternatives, such as meat, eggs, chicken, and foods that make you feel full while again loading your body with beneficial nutrients.

When you are shopping, avoid shopping for processed foods or candy and sweets. They are full of artificial sweeteners and sugars that will cause you to exceed the physiological recommended carb limit with just a few bites.

Instead, you can opt for fruits. They are like candy from nature; however, be careful to choose foods with a low glycemic index, such as avocados, strawberries, berries, peaches, etc. Decrease your intake of fruits that have a high glycemic index, such as bananas.

Energy drinks, sports drinks, and fizzy drinks are dangerous not only to your diet but also to your health. If you love having fluids, it is an excellent option to blend some low-glycemic fruits and make a smoothie or drink plenty of water or skimmed milk. It is much healthier in terms of managing weight and promoting your overall health to drink fruit smoothies, as they contain lots of nutrients and vitamins that are beneficial for your overall health. Sweetened tea, coffee with sugar, flavored coffee or chocolate drinks, and energy drinks are some of the worst options you can have as they are full of sugars. Instead, you can have black coffee with low-fat milk.

Snacking can be one of the subconscious ways to load up on sugars without even realizing it. All those chips, crisps, and crackers are full of artificial flavors and refined, processed sugars. A healthy option is to snack on celery or carrots. Snacking on cucumber bites with tahini sauce is a very healthy low-carb snack option full of fibers beneficial for your colon health and helps lower your cholesterol.

Meat, fish and seafood, chicken, and eggs are proteins that are good for you. Keep the meat low in fat. If you are eating poultry, trim the skin off. Moreover, it is better to go for plant-based protein as you will get more nutrients and fibers that are not present in animal products. Try to avoid fried meat or meat with high-fat cuts; for example, ribs, pork, bacon, added cheese, or deep-fried fish are all unhealthy options due to the added unhealthy fats.

Fats, oils, and sweets are some of the favorite food of many people; however, you need to be extra careful about your choice of fats from natural sources; for example, vegetables, nut seeds, and avocados are very healthy. However, try to keep to small proportions of foods that also give you Omega-3 fatty acids, such as salmon, tuna, and mackerel. Other healthy options are grape seed oil, olive oil, and plant-based oils. For healthy options, try to avoid anything that has trans-fat in it and also avoid partially-hydrogenated fats.

It can be challenging initially, but you have to skip desserts such as ice cream and any sugar-loaded food. You can keep those options as a reward on your cheat day. If you are craving a dessert, you can try dipping some low glycemic index fruits in some heavy whipping cream or cream cheese while topping it off with berries. This is a very healthy way to stay low in carbs while also gaining fat, which you need. If you absolutely must have chocolates, it is a much healthier option to go for dark chocolate; however, try not to do that often.

The Lean and Green diet provides convenience to people as it is a convenient meal replacement that removes the guesswork for many of its dieters. The Lean and Green Diet, was developed by Dr. William Vitale and encouraged people to eat healthy to achieve sustainable weight loss.

Under this diet regimen, dieters follow a weight loss plan, including five Fuelings a day and one Lean and Green meal. One of the popular diet plans that Lean and Green offers is the 5&1 plan designed for rapid weight loss. With this diet plan, users need to eat five of Lean and Green's Fuelings and one Lean and Green meal daily.

With the meal replacement and Lean and Green meals, this diet is perfect for people who want to lose weight and wish to transition from their old unhealthy habits to a healthier one. Thus, this is perfect for people who suffer from gout, diabetes, and people in their senior years.

Because it is a commercial diet, it has been subjected to different studies involving its efficacy. Studies have noted that people can lose weight in as little as 8 weeks; therefore, this is one of the most efficient diet regimens there is, as people can adapt and eventually embrace it as part of their lifestyles. Read on to learn about the Lean and Green diet.

Foods to Avoid When on Low-Carb

Beverages That Are Sweetened with Sugar

These beverages are some of the worst choices to obtain. This is because they are very high in carbs. For example, a 12-ounce can of soda has roughly 38 grams of carbs. The same applies to sweetened iced tea or sweetened lemonade as they contain about 35 grams of carbs per serving.

Trans Fats

These are fats that are made by adding hydrogen to unsaturated fatty acids to stabilize them. Examples of trans fats can be found in margarine and frozen dinners. Besides, many food companies add trans fats to the muffins and baked goods for better taste and extend their expiry date.

Trans fats do not directly affect raising your blood glucose levels; however, they increase your insulin resistance and promote the accumulation of fat. Don't disturb your fat metabolism and decrease your good cholesterol because this has the indirect effect of losing control of your weight management.

Pasta, Rice and White Bread

All these foods are rich in carbohydrates and quickly get digested to release lots of glucose into the blood. Besides, these foods are low in nutrients and have very little fiber, so the overall nutritional value is almost insignificant. Food rich in fiber is essential for controlling weight, cholesterol levels, and blood pressure; therefore, the main bulk of your food should be dedicated to foods that are high in fiber.

Fruit-Flavored Yogurt

Simple plain yogurt is a very healthy option. On the contrary, yogurt that is fruit-flavored is entirely different. They are often made from non-fat milk, and they are loaded with carbohydrates and sugars. One serving of fruit-flavored yogurt has about 47 grams of carbohydrates in the form of sugar. Instead of choosing yogurt that is flavored and rich in sugars, opt for simple, sugar-free, whole milk yogurt, which is helpful for your gut health and helps lose weight.

Fruits to Avoid

Grapes

A single grape contains 1 gram of carbohydrates, which means if you eat 30 grapes, you are easily eating 30 grams of carbs. And you can eat the same number of berries or strawberries while having significantly less amount of carbohydrates.

Cherries

They are super delicious; that is why it is hard to stop eating them once you have started; however, they are very rich in sugars and can cause your blood sugar to spike quickly.

Pineapple

When fresh and ripe, they can have a very high glycemic index. If you must eat pineapples, try to have a small serving of about half a cup and eat it with low-fat food, for example, Greek yogurt. Don't eat canned pineapple, as they are sweetened with unhealthy sugars.

Mango

These are super delicious foods; however, one single mango has about 30 grams of carbohydrates and nearly 25 grams of sugars. A riper and softer mango will have a higher glycemic index, while a firm mango will have a relatively lower glycemic index.

Banana

It is one of those too sweet yet very delicious foods. A medium-sized banana has about the same ounces of carbohydrates, which is double of any other fruit.

If you must have a banana, try to have half a serving and refrigerate the rest of it for another time.

Dried fruits seem harmless, especially when you add them to your food; however, two tablespoons of dried raisins have a similar amount of carbohydrates as just one cup of blueberries or another small piece of another fruit. That is because the water content has dried out, and their sugars have significantly been concentrated. Remove dried fruits from your diet and add fresh ones to your diet instead.

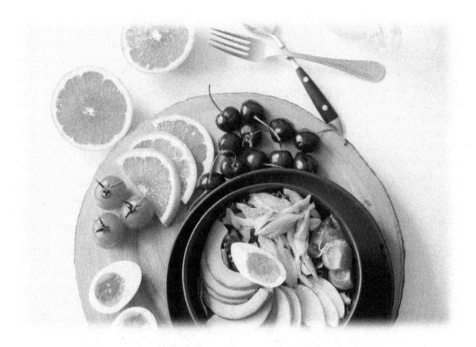

General Guide When Choosing Food to Eat

No matter what kind of diet you are attempting to follow, it is not correct to eliminate an entire food group. While on low carb, you can try minimizing your intake of starch and sugars but don't fall prey to the mistake of eliminating starch as your body needs carbs. Instead, you must choose wisely between the various food options in each category to ensure that you ingest the best and most suitable food type from each category and avoid the ones that will worsen your condition.

The goal of controlling your food with Lean and Green is eating food that will not increase your blood glucose levels higher than usual. At the same time, it needs to be food that makes you feel full and keeps hunger at bay; besides, specific food categories can promote your health and provide you with nutritional elements that can help you fight off your weight increase and protect you from its complications.

Low-Starch Food

Whole grains, for example, oatmeal, quinoa, and brown rice, are preferred and healthier than white rice, white flour or processed grains, macaroni, etc.

Baked sweet potato provides a low-carb option in contrast to regular potatoes, such as French fries. Other items that are high in carbs include white bread and white flour etc. Instead, opt for whole-grain foods that have very little added sugar or none at all.

Non-Starchy Vegetables

One of the healthiest options if you have diabetes is to include a couple of servings of non-starchy vegetables per day. There is very little chance that you could go wrong with overeating non-starchy vegetables; that is because they have a deficient calorific intake.

Non-starchy vegetables are vegetables that contain a small number of carbohydrates. This is typically about 5 grams or less of carbohydrates per 100 grams of serving non-starchy vegetables.

It should be your goal throughout your day that you have at least five portions of fruit and vegetables, and out of those 5, it is best to have at least three of them that are non-starchy vegetables.

There are several reasons why non-starchy vegetables are very healthy options for low carb. The foremost reason is that they are deficient in carbs. Other causes include how non-starchy vegetables are very nutritious. They are full of vitamins and minerals as well as other critical nutrients such as phytochemicals. Besides being vegetables, they are a crucial source of dietary fiber. Dietary fiber will help you digest food properly, and it also plays an essential role in lowering your cholesterol levels. Overall, dietary fiber is a crucial nutrient to include in your diet.

Non-starchy vegetables are also rich in vitamins and minerals such as vitamin A, vitamin C, and vitamin K. Vitamin C helps promote your immunity and protect your cells from oxidative damage.

A good source of non-starchy vegetables containing vitamin C are peppers, sprouts, and broccoli. You can easily add peppers to your salad or main dish. Steamed broccoli is also a very healthy option to add to your main dish, serve alongside salmon, or add to your veggie pan salad.

Vitamin E is also helpful in boosting your immune system; it is also essential for your eye health and skin. Carrots, kale, and spinach are options rich in vitamin E that you can easily add to your food. Below are some examples of non-starchy vegetables:

- **Leafy vegetables:** Kale, lettuce, spinach, watercress, cabbage, and Brussel sprouts
- **Root vegetables:** Carrot, turnip, and radishes
- **Squashes:** Cucumber, squash, courgette, and pumpkin
- **Stalk vegetables:** Asparagus, leeks, spring onions, and celery
- **Others:** Broccoli, bean sprouts, mushroom, cauliflower, peppers, and tomato

Vegetables are your best friends. When eaten raw or even when steamed, roasted, or grilled, fresh vegetables can be a very healthy low-carb option. The same applies to frozen vegetables that are lightly cooked. Always opt for low-sodium or unsalted canned vegetables. Canned vegetables with lots of added sodium are not a healthy option.

It is also counterproductive if you eat veggies cooked with lots of butter cheese or a high carb source. If you have hypertension or other diabetes and metabolic syndrome complications, you need to limit your sodium intake, including pickles, etc.

Fatty Fish

Fatty fish are one of the most consistent diet recommendations when it comes to fending off diseases. Some examples are herring, salmon anchovies, mackerel, and sardine.

Salmon contains Omega-3 fatty acids, which have a profound positive effect on your heart health. Taking care of and promoting your heart health helps against the increased risk of heart disease and stroke that people with diabetes are faced with. Studies have shown that several inflammatory markers had dropped when fatty fish was consumed 5 to 7 days per week for about 8 weeks. In addition to all that, it contains high-quality protein and is low in carbs; therefore, it is perfect for maintaining normal blood glucose sugars after meals.

Dairy

Dairy food is a vital food category and with various choices available for you to pick from. Studies have shown that milk product consumption and total dairy products have been associated with a reduced risk of developing type 2 diabetes. It is also protective for those who have prediabetes. The studies were conducted on items from the dairy group, including whole milk and yogurt and total dairy consumption.

Examples of dairy food include milk, yogurt, cream, butter, and cheese. Unsweetened dairy products can be a very healthy choice for those who wish to follow a low-carb diet. There are numerous benefits of dairy foods, as they are a good source of protein, calcium, and vitamin B12. The National Osteoporosis Society recommends that a daily intake of 700 milligrams of calcium is required for adults to maintain healthy bones and other functions that depend on calcium.

Vitamin B12 is an essential source for the nervous system. People with diabetes are at risk of complications of neuropathy that affects the peripheral nerves. Vitamin B12 helps protect against some of the complications of diabetes concerning the nerves. The protein in milk is also essential for muscle repair and growth. The recommended daily intake of calcium can be achieved by just a pint of milk along with another source that includes food such as beans, fish with edible bones like sardines and salmon, and dark green vegetables, for example, kale and broccoli.

For dairy, opt for low-fat dairy; if you want to have high-fat or full-fat dairy, do so but in small proportions. The best choices are skimmed milk, low-fat yogurt, and low-fat or non-fat sour cream or cottage cheese. Some of the worst options are whole milk, regular yogurt, regular sour cream, cottage cheese, and ice cream, etc.

Beans and Pulses

Beans, pulses, lentils, peas, chickpeas, and runner beans are all examples of non-animal sources of protein that can be very beneficial to people with diabetes.

Soya Beans have been included among this group, and it has been supported with research indicating that the consumption of soya beans increases insulin sensitivity and reduces the risk of developing type 2 diabetes.

Adding beans to your salads is a good option for increasing your protein intake.

Fruits to Eat on Low-Carb Diet

Like vegetables, fruits are among the healthiest food groups that you can add to your diet. They are rich in nutrients, especially vitamin C, which helps keep your cells healthy. In addition to the minerals, we also have fiber that aids digestion reducing cholesterol levels. Different fruits have a different combination of vitamins and minerals; for example, grapefruits can be rich in vitamin A and potassium; they can also be rich in vitamin K and manganese.

While fruits have dense nutrients, fiber, and antioxidants, it is important to remember that certain foods have a high glycemic index and can increase your blood sugar levels; therefore, it is essential to be mindful about the types of fruits you eat and when.

Watermelon and Dates

Avoid processed foods, such as apple sauce that have had their fiber removed. If you have a sweet tooth, fruits can be an optimum way to satisfy your desires without compromising your health. Since

LEAN AND GREEN DIET COOKBOOK

fruits are high in nutrients and low in fat and sodium, they are optimum if you have obesity or hypertension.

One serving of fruit is a medium-sized fruit that is the size of the piece or a cup of smaller fruits such as berries. You should avoid it, but processed fruits have only half a cup of additives to fulfill the serving size.

Apples

An apple is a versatile fruit that you can snack on raw or cook with some flavoring such as cinnamon or ginger to make a delicious dessert. You can also stuff your apples with some crushed nuts such as walnuts or pecans.

Avocados

Avocados are very high in healthy fats, which are the monounsaturated fats that are beneficial to your body. Avocados are a tasty option to add to your main dish; slice them along with some salmon or make guacamole. They're straightforward to prepare or include in any of your dishes.

Berries

Berries are very delicious and versatile fruits. There are strawberries, blueberries, blackberries, etc. There are a lot of things that you can do with berries; for example, you can eat them raw, or you can make them into a smoothie. You can always add various berries to most of your breakfast or snacks, for example, making an oatmeal breakfast or adding mixed berries to your fresh whipped cream or frozen yogurt. They are also rich in antioxidants and very low in calories. They help fight inflammation and other diseases such as cancer.

Citrus Fruits

They are also useful for boosting your immunity; they are loaded with vitamin C. One orange contains all the amount of vitamin C that you require in a day. Since immunity is an issue with people with diabetes, adding citrus foods to your diet is very healthy and a useful low carb option. You can add lemons to your seafood, sauces, or even to your iced water or tea. You can simply make lemons or oranges into a refreshing cold drink. The folate and potassium in oranges help you equalize your blood pressure if you suffer from hypertension. Citrus foods also include grapefruits as well as oranges and lemons.

38 | P a g .

Peaches

They are juicy and delicious fragrant foods containing lots of nutrients such as vitamins A and C and fiber and minerals such as potassium. They are easy to add to your yogurt or spice them up with some cinnamon or ginger. You can also flavor your tea with peach instead of sugar for a healthy twist on your drinks.

Pears are also tasty treats that you can add up to your salad or snack on. They are rich in fiber and are a good source of vitamin K.

Kiwi is a slightly citrus fruit that is rich in fiber and vitamin C as well as potassium. One large kiwi contains about 13 grams of carbohydrates, which is low carb, making it a delicious yet very healthy option to add to your diet.

Lean Meat

A source of protein that is low in fat and low in calories is lean meat. That means the red meat such as pork chops trimmed with fat or skinless chicken or turkey.

Lean meat is a nutritional protein source for promoting cell health and repair—while also being a low-carb and low-fat option. Poultry is also a rich source of vitamin B3, B6 choline, and selenium. Vitamin B3, which is known as niacin, helps with stress and sex hormones. Erectile dysfunction and stress are an issue for those who have diabetes, and having food with vitamin B3 become very beneficial for people with diabetes. Niacin helps with promoting the nerve functions and can reduce inflammation. Selenium has strong antioxidant properties that help with controlling inflammation and protecting the cells. Selenium also has a role in promoting the immune system, which is very beneficial to people with diabetes.

Red meat is also a rich source of protein, iron, zinc, and vitamin B. Iron is essential for your red blood cells to transport oxygen, as healthy cells require a constant supply of oxygen. Anemia, which is a deficiency in RBCs (Red Blood Cells), can occur due to a lack of iron—which is a condition that could easily be avoided by eating adequate amounts of this mineral. Iron can also be found in dark, green, leafy plants and beans; iron from greens are the best source.

Zinc is also a mineral needed by the body for the synthesis of DNA. It also has a role in helping the immune system to function properly. You can also find zinc in fish eggs and beans, although zinc is better absorbed from fish and meat sources.

Red meat is rich in vitamin B6 and B12. Both help promote the immune system, regeneration, and protection of the nervous system. One medication that some people with diabetes take, known as metformin, causes an increased drop in vitamin B12. Therefore, it becomes necessary to compensate for vitamin B loss from sources such as red meat.

Eggs

Be mindful about the number of eggs you consume, as they can easily raise your cholesterol levels. If you're going to eat an egg, it is preferred to boil and consume the whole egg, as the benefits of eggs line in the nutrients inside rather than the whites. It is a debate whether eggs are helpful or not to people with diabetes due to their low carb content; however, consuming an excessive amount of eggs is associated with increased cholesterol levels. Moreover, apart from being rich in cholesterol, eggs are dense in nutrients, as they have essential fatty acids, proteins, and vitamin D.

Nuts

Nuts that reduce bad cholesterol are very effective because they protect people with diabetes from complications of the narrowing of arteries.

Consuming cashews is very beneficial to lower your blood pressure and decrease the risk of heart disease. They are also low in calories; therefore, they have no negative effect on your blood glucose level. They are also low in fat, so they do not affect your weight negatively. You can have about a handful of cashews every day for the maximum benefit.

Peanuts are rich in fiber and protein, and therefore, they are a beneficial option for people who have diabetes. You can have up to 25 to 30 peanuts every day. You can also roast them. They can control your blood glucose levels.

They are loaded with energy; however, they are good sources of protein and a good source of healthy fats, making you feel full for a long time; therefore, curbing the urge to snack. A study performed showed that eating pistachios was very beneficial to people who have diabetes. Avoid salted pistachios.

Walnuts are high in calories; however, they do not affect your body weight. They have numerous nutritional benefits. Consuming walnuts daily can help in weight loss due to their low-carb content and their possession of substances that activate the fat-burning pathways. They also provoke fasting glucose, which helps you avoid obesity as a complication of diabetes. The high-calorie content helps your body by providing it with energy to don't feel like eating a lot and gaining weight.

Almonds control the blood glucose level and are very beneficial to people with diabetes because they reduce the oxidative stress that affects cells in diabetics. They are also rich in magnesium. You should avoid salted almonds, but you can also soak them in water overnight to eat them fresh the next day.

How to Tackle Low-Carb Eating?

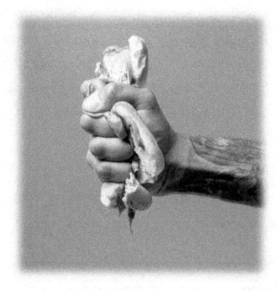

We don't eat just to relieve physical hunger. For warmth, stress reduction, or to reward oneself, many of us often turn to food. And we prefer to reach out for fast food, candy, and other soothing yet harmful things when we do. When you feel sad, you may reach for a cup of ice cream, order a pizza if you are bored and lonely, or stop by the drive-through after a long day at work.

Emotional eating involves food to help oneself feel better, rather than the stomach, to meet emotional needs. Comfort eating, sadly, doesn't cure emotional issues. Probably, it generally makes you feel worse. Afterward, the initial mental struggle not only persists, but you feel bad about binge eating as well.

It isn't always a negative thing to sometimes use eating as a pick-me-up, a treat, or rejoice. But when food is the main emotional coping method, you get trapped in an addictive loop where the actual feeling or concern is never tackled. Your first instinct is to open the fridge anytime you are depressed, frustrated, furious, sad, tired, or bored.

How you consume is just as or even more significant than what you consume. In emotional overeating, the overall amount of food you consume, your disposition toward eating, how you manage your snacks and meals, and your personal food choices may play a far greater role than the actual foods you want to consume. Take time to evaluate your eating habits, understand more about regular eating vs. emotional eating, and build different self-help methods to resolve both your mental and physical food relationships. Start practicing saying "no," not just to harmful foods but also to circumstances that undermine your attempts to build healthier dietary patterns that are emotionally mindful.

When you're emotionally at the weakest place, the worst food cravings strike. When experiencing a tough situation, feeling depressed, or even feeling bored, you may look to food for warmth—consciously or subconsciously. Comfort eating will undermine your attempts to lose weight. It also contributes to excessive consumption, particularly too much of high-calorie, fatty and sugary desserts. The positive news is that you may take action to retake control of your dietary behaviors and get back on board with your weight reduction plans if you're susceptible to emotional eating.

Recognize Addictive Behavior

Study studies have been dedicated to the issue of food addiction for years, whether or not anyone may be addicted to certain foods, specifically those created with processed goods such as white flour, sugar, salt, and fat, and whether, in turn, these foods were accountable for such habits of bingeing and excessive consumption. As it could not be proved that food itself became addictive, scientists started to look at the habits' addictive features. Addiction components include addictive behavior involvement (such as overeating), lack of control, behavioral preoccupation (eating), having only brief gratification, and permanent detrimental effects (becoming unhealthy or obese from overeating).

Separate Emotional Signals from Hunger Signals

The distinction between feeding in reaction to appetite and feeding in reaction to emotion may be challenging to perceive and recognize. Through feeding mindfully and paying attention to hunger cues, learn to distinguish the two types of feeding and self-regulate your food intake. Practice evaluating your hunger: Exactly how hungry are you on a scale of 1 to 10? If you don't feel hungry or you're only a little hungry, anywhere between one and four, you should rank it. Wait until you hit five, very hungry (but don't let yourself get too hungry to the extent you overeat).

Develop a Schedule

Eating regularly scheduled meals and scheduled snacks for certain persons will deter overeating if you keep to the routine. On the other side, since they lead to random feeding and bingeing, erratic eating patterns typically mean disaster. Generally speaking, at various hours of the day, most people plan three courses and one or two snacks or "micro meals." Typically, true hunger comes in about three hours after the last meal. A tiny snack might be enough at that moment, depending on your eating patterns and the time of day; if not, you get a signal that it's time for your next meal.

Change the Eating Patterns

Some research has shown that missing food, consuming late at night, and other irregular eating habits may contribute to weight gain for some individuals. It doesn't imply that as soon as you wake up the next morning, you can or should have breakfast, nor does it imply that you shouldn't consume something at night. However, it might be time to follow a different pattern if eating habits don't help you shed weight or manage over-eating. Short-term research has also shown that consuming the main meal at noon (for lunch) will promote weight reduction and weight management, rather than later in the day or what might be deemed usual dinner time.

Find Different Ways to Satisfy Your Emotions

You would not be able to regulate your food habits for too long if you don't know how to handle your feelings in a manner that doesn't rely on food. Diets too frequently fail because they provide rational dietary guidance that only works if the food patterns are deliberately managed when feelings derail the system, expecting an instant payoff with food, so it doesn't work.

In order to prevent emotional feeding, you must find other avenues to satisfy yourself psychologically. It's not enough to grasp the emotional eating cycle or even to recognize their causes, even though it's a big first step. For emotional satisfaction, you need substitutes for food that you can resort to.

Several other alternatives to comfort eating are given here:

- Call somebody who always helps you feel good, whether you're sad or lonely, interact with your cat or dog, or glance at a childhood picture or special photo album.
- Release your inner tension if you're restless by listening to your favorite tune, holding a tension ball, or enjoying a fast stroll.

- Give yourself a hot cup of tea if you're tired, take a nap, light some scented candles, or get yourself in a heated blanket.
- Read a good novel, watch a television show, wander in nature, or switch to a hobby that you love (woodworking, guitar playing, playing basketball, jigsaw puzzles, etc.) if you're bored.

Get Social Support

If needed, a community of friends and family, including clinical support in the form of a psychologist or mentor, may be as vital to your progress as your own encouragement and actions. Many that care for your well-being will assist by supporting you, exchanging suggestions for healthy foods, acknowledging the social foundations of your unhealthy eating problems, and maybe even helping to solve any of the mental conditions that affect your emotional eating. Surround yourself with friends who are able to lend an ear, give support and inspiration, or maybe join in as buddies for dining, walking, or exercising.

THE PROTEIN BALANCE

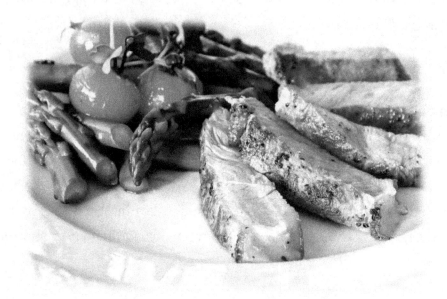

The human body requires fuel in order to provide energy for our cells. The three fuel sources in food consist of protein, carbohydrates, and fat. After these are eaten, the digestion system breaks them down into purer forms of energy, including amino acids from protein, glucose from carbohydrates, and fatty acids from fat. The human body is capable of surviving without consumption of carbohydrates/glucose, as it is capable of transmuting other sources of fuel into any glucose the cells might need in a process known as gluconeogenesis. However, the same is not true for amino acids and fatty acids. There are certain types of amino acids and fatty acids that the human body requires but is unable to produce on its own. This means that we must consume these fatty acids and amino acids in our diet.

The protein, or amino acids, are used by your body in order to repair damaged tissues, replace old tissues, build muscle, and fight off infections. Thankfully, most people are able to consume protein in the required ranges—neither too much nor too little—without much effort. As long as they eat a few protein-rich ingredients daily, they can achieve the correct amount of protein. The same is not true for people with kidney diseases, who have to be more diligent in managing how much protein they do or don't consume in their diet.

When a person consumes too much protein, it can cause a buildup of excess waste in their blood. As you know, kidney disease results in the kidneys being unable to filter the blood, resulting in excess waste buildup. This means that if a person consumes too much protein when they have kidney disease, they will only be worsening the problem of waste overabundance, and their kidneys will not be capable of handling it. Therefore, it is imperative that people with kidney disease are aware of the amount of protein they consume and that they don't put more than necessary in their meals.

Without amino acids, the body would be incapable of fighting off infections, healing from injuries, and halting excessive bleeding. We would be unable to have any muscle, as well, which would be deadly as the human heart is a muscle itself. This is why it is important to maintain adequate protein intake in your diet. For an average person, protein between forty and sixty-five grams daily is ideal.

There are two types of protein you will consume in your daily diet, which are animal-based proteins and plant-based proteins. A person can choose to consume either a combination of both animal and plant proteins or solely plant-based proteins if they are vegan.

Animal-based proteins are simple to add to your diet, as they contain all of the amino acid building blocks your body requires. This means all you have to worry about is consuming the correct amount of protein. The amount and types of fat found within animal-based protein varies based on the source of the ingredients. For example, steak contains much more fat than chicken breasts. Some animal-based proteins are also higher in saturated fats, which are a less healthy option for heart health. When trying to consume low-saturated fat options for optimal heart health, people typically choose poultry, fish, and reduced-fat dairy options.

Plant-based sources of protein are more versatile in the amino acids they contain. While animal-based proteins contain all the essential amino acids humans require, the variety of amino acids found in most plant-based ingredients is usually reduced. For this reason, if you are relying on plant-based proteins, you will need to ensure you are consuming all nine essential amino acids, which include:

- Lysine

- Isoleucine

- Histidine

- Leucine

- Valine

- Threonine

- Phenylalanine

- Methionine

- Tryptophan

While there are twenty types of amino acids in all, these nine are the most essential to consume in our diets. For this reason, whenever an ingredient contains all nine essential amino acids, it is classified as a complete source of protein. While animal-based products are complete sources of protein, not all plant-based ingredients are. Thankfully, there are still complete sources of plant-based protein, which are important to know about if you are consuming most or all of your protein from plant-based sources. Some examples of complete sources of protein include quinoa, soy, buckwheat, rice paired with beans, and chia seeds. While these are complete sources of protein, you can still get additional amino acids from nuts, grains, lentils, beans, seeds, and vegetables. If people plan their plant-based diet carefully, they can ensure that they are consuming the correct amount of protein needed for their kidney health and the correct amino acids. Plant-based protein sources are also beneficial as they are low in saturated fat, high in fiber, and high in nutrients.

While the exact amount of protein you will need to consume will vary based on the factors we have previously mentioned, frequently, people who are in stages one through three of chronic kidney disease are recommended twelve to fifteen percent of their calorie intake to be protein. If a person is in stage four of chronic kidney disease, this percentage is further reduced, often to being around ten percent of a person's daily caloric intake.

Americans are used to enjoying large servings of protein-rich ingredients, such as meat, fish, and dairy. This can lead to confusion about what you can eat if you have to limit these ingredients to such a degree. This is especially confusing when you consider the fact that you must consume enough calories daily to prevent excessive weight loss and muscle waste. Thankfully, there are healthy ingredients that you can add to your meals to increase their nutrition and bulk up calories. One easy way to do this is by adding olive oil or avocado oil to your meals. These two oils are high in some of the healthiest fatty acids and are high in calories, allowing people to bulk up their calorie content easily.

The exact cause for this improvement with plant-based proteins has not been confirmed. However, there are multiple factors that could be responsible. First, plant-based ingredients are often high in phytonutrients and antioxidants, which have been shown to fight disease and improve overall health. Second, the consumption of these ingredients seems to reduce the production of uremic toxins, which are a type of toxin that is known to worsen the progression of chronic kidney disease and cardiovascular disease.

The third cause of this benefit could lie in the consumption of phosphorus. This mineral, which is known to become overly concentrated in the blood of chronic kidney disease patients, is found in both plant-based and animal-based protein sources. However, the difference is that phosphorus has a different bioavailability rate in both of these sources. While the phosphorus found in animal-based proteins are easily absorbed by the body, the same is not true for plant-based protein sources.

Is Lean and Green Diet Going to Help You Lose Weight?

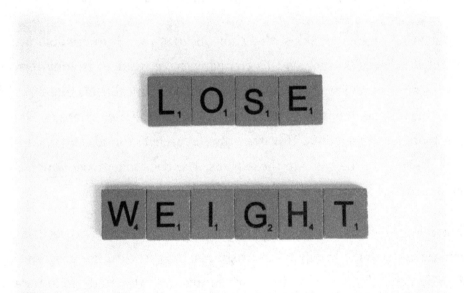

How much weight you lose following the Lean and Green diet plans depends on factors such as your starting weight and age, and how well you conform to the plan, and how involved you are.

Lean and Green reflects the group of coaches and specific lifestyle brand, introduced in 2017. Previous experiments have been carried out using the old products and not the current Lean and Green products. Although the Lean and Green goods are a new line, the parent company told "U.S. News" that they have the same macronutrient profile and are also comparable to the original products as well. Therefore, when testing this diet, we assume that the following studies are important. There has been no literature conducted directly on the label Lean and Green.

The studies were limited, with many dropouts, as is true with most diets. Short term, it seems difficult not to lose at least a few pounds; you consume half the calories that other adults consume. Studies appear to back it up. Long term views are less optimistic. Look at the data in more detail here:

A 2017 study funded by a well-known company found that by their final visit (anywhere from 4 to 24 weeks later), more than 70% of overweight adults who entered this program and received one-on-one therapeutic support lost more than 5% of their body mass.

A 2016 research—partially funded by a nutritional product company that and published in the journal Obesity—found that obese adults lost 8.8% of their body weight with these products and Lean and Green -style coaching after 12 weeks, and 12.1 percent of their body weight if they took phentermine at the same time—a weight loss medication that can minimize food cravings.

A research published by "Johns Hopkins Medicine" in 2015 found no credible evidence that most commercial weight loss services, such as this company, have resulted in long-term weight loss for individuals. The researchers reviewed articles on randomized clinical trials that lasted for 12 weeks or more. In trials lasting 4 to six months, participants in low-calorie meal plans, such as this company, lost more weight than nonparticipants. However, the researchers found only one long-term analysis, which at 12 months showed little value to those plans. The researchers also found that the very low-calorie systems carried higher risks of complications, including gallstones.

A 2015 research released in the "Annals of Internal Medicine" reviewed 45 trials, including this company, of generic and patented weight-loss programs. Very low-calorie programs, culminated in a weight loss of 4% greater than therapy for four months. But the study found some of this effect lessened after six months of reporting.

A 2015 research in the "Diet Journal" looked at the charts of 310 overweight and obese clients who followed the "Achieve Plan" and found which participants—who remained on the plan—lost an average of around 24 pounds by week 12 and 35 pounds by week 24. Participants lost more fat than lean muscle no matter their age or gender.

A small research, sponsored and planned by this company and published in "Nutrition Journal" in 2010, has randomly allocated 90 obese adults to either the 5&1 plan or a calorie-restricted diet based on government guidelines. Those in the well-known company category had lost a total of 30 pounds after 16 weeks—compared to the other 14 pounds in th group. But 24 weeks later, dieters on this program had regained more than 10 pounds after dieters had increased their calories, while the others had put back on about 2 pounds. The first category group at week 40 had less body fat and more muscle mass at the start but did not outperform the control group. Almost half of the first group and more than half of the control group ended up dropping out.

A study of 119 overweight or obese Type 2 diabetics, published in the "Diabetes Educator" in 2008, randomly assigned dietitians to a diabetic plan or a diet based on "American Diabetes Association (ADA)" guidelines. After 34 weeks, the well-known company group had lost a total of 10 1/2 pounds but had recovered all but 3 pounds after 86 weeks. At week 34, the diabetics on the ADA-based diet lost a total of 3 pounds; after 86 weeks, they'd gained it all back plus a pound. The dropout rate was almost 80%.

What Do You get from These Lean and Green Diet Recipes?

If you find yourself going off and on a rollercoaster eating habit, you should definitely try out the recipes outlined in this book. Lean and Green diet comes with the structure and organization needed to get you off on a good start and take you to your desired destination if well-adhered to. Anyway, my friends' account simply portrays that some discipline is, of course, required. Even if you're an emotional eater or a binge eater, the Lean and Green diet encourages you to exercise a bit of control.

The diet is a high-protein diet that typically makes up about 10–35% of your daily calorie intake. The protein serves as a carb alternative when your body needs energy. On average, your calorie intake per day may hover around 800–1,000 as the Lean and Green diet relies on the intense restriction of calories and active promotion of weight loss. The Calories of most of the Fuelings is around 100–110 each.

Lean and Green diets encourage you to do away with junk by eating nutrition-rich Fuelings and making your own food based on a healthy template. If you are often too busy to cook, the diet allows for a varying degree of flexibility when it comes to preparing your own meal, as well as a complementary degree of pre-packaged foods or Fuelings to go with your cooking timetable. In essence, following the program is a no brainer as a structure that has been provided for you. For individuals seeking to achieve weight loss through healthy eating, the recipes included serve just that purpose, but your eating plan will depend on whether you're watching your weight or trying to reduce your weight. Whatever the case, the plans are simple and detailed. The coaching and community support help you adhere to the structure of the program.

In case you didn't know, the "Fuelings" are the features that make Lean and Green recipes stand out among many other weight loss programs. The Fuelings are made without artificial additives, colors, or sweeteners. In addition to that, their "select" line is preservative-free. Although the meals are mostly pre-packaged, especially for the first two levels, they still do not contain any stimulants and no wacky pills or supplements. The emphasis is instead placed on regular eating of small portions of meals and snacks each day.

Previous studies by the team of this company showed that the Lean and Green diet might help improve blood pressure in obese people. This is due to the reduction in weight and reduced sodium intake. Research shows that high sodium levels aggravate the risk of high blood pressure in persons with underlying health conditions, especially salt-sensitive individuals. Lean and Green meal plans generally provide less than 2,300 milligrams of sodium throughout the day. However, this may vary when it comes to the Lean and Green meals, in which case you're at liberty to choose between low and high sodium options. Also, the recipes are simple and easy to make, so you don't have to worry about spending too much time in the kitchen.

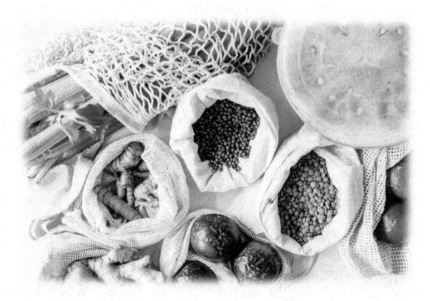

What to Buy

Eggs: Eggs are the best source of protein. All kinds of eggs are okay to eat. Normally, egg whites should be preferred, but yolks are fine too.

Chicken Breasts or Cutlets (Skinless): Chicken, like eggs, is a rich source of protein. Buy a good-quality, inexpensive, and lean chicken. You can cook this in a variety of ways. Given that chicken is perishable, always buy it fresh and use it immediately.

Ground Turkey (Lean): Although ground turkey is a bit more expensive, it is a good change when you get bored with eating chicken; you can rely on turkey as a rich source of protein. Once again, you should always buy a fresh turkey and use it immediately.

Steak: Avoid steak if you are on a very strict diet. If not, then you should not miss steak, as it is a good source of protein and fat. Only buy fresh and lean steak.

Mignon Filet: This is very expensive but tasty as well. Buy it occasionally to treat your palate.

Buffalo: This is definitely the most expensive meat on this list. Only buy fresh and lean buffalo meat.

Flounder: Flounder is an inexpensive fish bread that also happens to be very tasty. Buy it fresh as opposed to the frozen variety, but when you have no option, you can go for the frozen ones.

Cod: This is another inexpensive breed of fish that is packed with proteins and is tasty as well.

Pollock: This is a type of lean fish. It is found easily in the seafood section of the supermarket.

Salmon: Salmon is famous for its protein richness and taste. It is also rather fatty, so eat it in moderation. Wild salmon is more expensive than bred salmon.

Tuna (canned): Canned tuna is once again a tasty, inexpensive, and lean fish. However, if you are on a low-sodium diet, you should avoid this fish or eat it in moderation. In addition, only buy fish that is canned in water and not in oil.

Turkey Bacon: Bacon is generally not allowed on a bodybuilding diet, so as a replacement, you should consider buying turkey bacon. Eat it sparingly—twice a month is more than enough as a treat for your taste buds.

Ground Beef (Lean): Buy good-quality, 90% lean beef. It is a high source of protein and can be consumed in the off-season.

Paneer: Paneer is a form of cottage cheese that is popular in the Indian subcontinent. It is slow-digesting, so you can feel full and satiated for a long time. It is versatile, and you can make a variety of things with it.

Pork Tenderloin: Buy good-quality, low-cost, lean tenderloins, as they are a great source of proteins.

Bass (Sea): This is expensive but tasty. You can eat it occasionally.

Swordfish: This is expensive but tasty. You can eat it occasionally.

What Not to Buy

Skinned Chicken: Only buy skinless chicken, as the chicken skin is full of unhealthy fats that are best avoided.

Breaded Chicken: The breadcrumbs add unnecessary carbs to your diet.

Deli Meat: This is full of additives and preservatives and is generally of low quality.

Bacon: As said earlier, avoid bacon. It is tasty but very fatty and, thus, can wreak havoc on your diet plan. This is not good for heart-related issues.

Ground Beef (Fatty): Lean ground beef should be preferred over fatty beef because, as the name suggests, regular beef contains high amounts of fats.

Fatty Cuts of Meat: Go for lean cuts of meats always. Regular cuts generally contain unnecessary fats that are not good for your diet.

Why Lean and Green Diet Rather Than Other Diet?

Calorie Restriction Impact

Despite the fact that Lean and Green 's eating routine arrangement stresses eating every now and again for the duration of the day—every one of its "Fuelings" just gives 110 calories. "Lean and Green" foods are additionally low in calories.

At the point when you're eating fewer calories, all in all, you may discover the arrangement leaves you ravenous and unsatisfied. You may feel all the more effectively exhausted and even crabby.

Weariness and Isolation at Mealtimes

Lean and Green 's dependence on meal substitutions can meddle with the social parts of getting ready and eating food.

Clients may think that it's clumsy or baffling to have a shake or bar at a family supper time or when feasting out with companions.

How It Compares with others

The Lean and Green diet can be more viable for fast weight reduction than different plans, basically in view of what a limited number of calories its Fuelings and Lean and Green meals give.

"U.S. News" and "World Report" positioned Lean and Green as the number 2 best eating routine for quick weight reduction (attached with "Atkins," "keto," and "Weight Watchers").

The 2019 "U.S. News" and "World Report Best Diets" positioned the Lean and Green Diet 31st in "Best Diets Overall" and gave it a general score of 2.7/5.

Lean and Green requires less "mental tumbling" than contenders like "Weight Watchers" (for which you need to gain proficiency with an arrangement of focuses) or "keto" (for which you should intently follow and evaluate macronutrients).

Lean and Green's instructing segment is similar to "Weight Watchers" and "Jenny Craig," the two of which urge members to select in for meetups to get social help.

The exceptionally handled nature of most nourishments you'll eat on the Lean and Green diet can be a drawback contrasted with the variety of new, entire nourishments you can eat on increasingly independently directed plans, for example, Atkins.

Calorie restriction is essential to weight reduction, and the 5&1 option is particularly conducive to shedding weight rapidly with an 800–1,000-calorie nutritional plan. Carbs also are stored low with a decent amount of protein per serving, which is right for effective weight reduction in maximum instances.

Plus, carb and calorie restriction have shown to have many health advantages, which include advanced glucose metabolism, adjustments in frame composition, reduced danger of cardiovascular chance elements, and other disorder chance elements as nicely.

But the 5&1 plan may not be for anyone, as dropping weight quickly and excessive calorie restriction can be damaging to your health, and also you virtually won't feel excellent at the same time as muscle loss is likewise an opportunity. 800–1,000 calories are a quite low standard. However, for weight loss, eating 800–1,000 calories can be safe and effective if no longer applied for extended periods.

Research suggests that too few calories can have an effect on metabolism over the years that could make you regain the weight.

But this will additionally be due to long term habits as there are also several different variables to recall in terms of the differences among people. Weight loss isn't continually easy, and retaining it off may be even more difficult; however, it requires everlasting lifestyle changes.

Lean and Green additionally recommends 30 minutes a day of exercise, which is likewise important for maintaining the weight off and maintaining proper health.

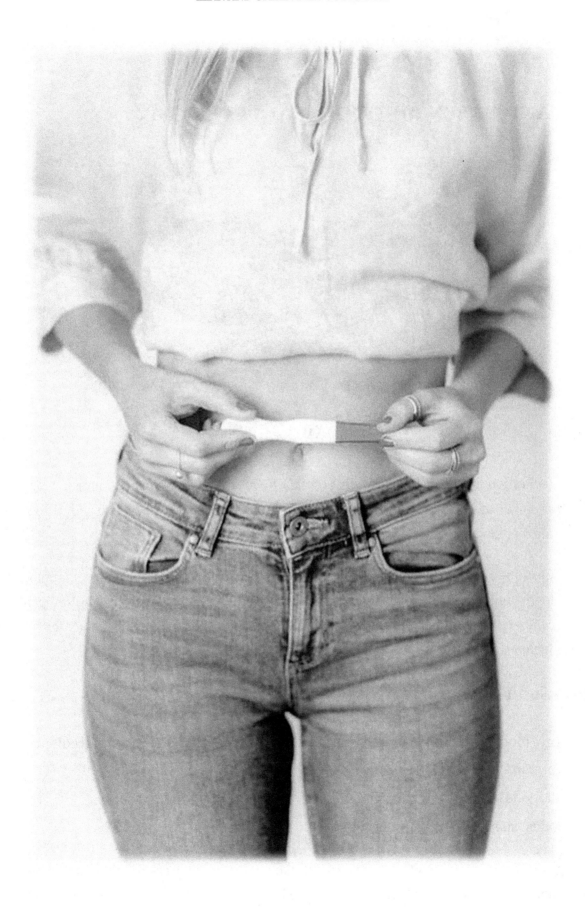

LEAN AND GREEN DIET IN 6 MEALS EVERYDAY

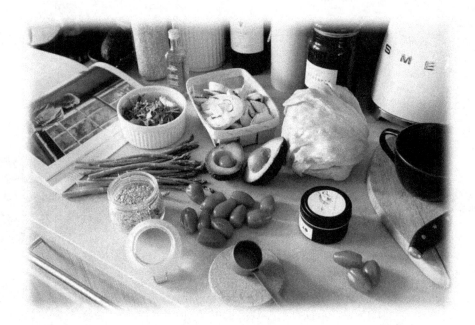

P reparation is the key to nearly all success! The more you can prepare yourself, your kitchen, and your meal planning before you try to start a diet, the more likely you will be to stick with the diet longer and see immediate results that last.

Cleaning out the kitchen is the first step in preparing for a diet. Before shopping for the foods and products, you'll need to start eating Keto, clear your refrigerator, pantry, and cabinets of anything that creates temptation, such as potato chips or ice cream. Other products include:

Processed Foods

- Any food that has sugar or starch listed within the first five ingredients on the nutrition label
- All foods and drinks containing high levels of carbohydrates or sugars
- Sodas, sugary drinks, and juices

Knowing how to shop is one of the most useful skills all diet followers develop as they adapt and become more familiar with how their body reacts to ketosis and what it requires to maintain the state.

Here is a look at a sample grocery shopping list put together based on the main ingredients that make up the foundation of a diet and the staples experts and veterans of the diet recommendations for beginners.

Understanding Portion Control

Before we dive into the lengthy details of what the Lean and Green diet really is and how it works, it is very important first to grasp the whole idea of portion control and the "six-small-frequent-meals" philosophy to lose weight. That is why this first chapter is a comprehensive introduction to the idea of eating smaller meals more frequently throughout the day. We'll start off by introducing the concept of portion control. This would be a great start for people who have never heard of it or never practiced this method of healthy eating and losing weight. Then, we'll get into the significance of it in our daily lives, i.e., why to practice it and what happens if we don't. After that, a section is dedicated to the very many benefits of controlling and limiting our food portions, along with the reasoning and principles behind the efficacy of six small meals per day. Towards the end, we'll touch upon a very important issue of emotional eating (also known as comfort eating). We'll discuss what it is and what are the different ways to actually practice it efficiently in order to shed pounds and be healthier. Finally, the very last section will entail some valuable and easy-to-follow tips and tricks to practice portion control for all of you who struggle with the issue.

What Is Portion Control?

Are you having difficulty reducing weight? Even if you make healthy lifestyle decisions like denying candy, exchanging French fries with a Caesar salad, and sweating crazy during the workouts? Do you keep on mounting the scale week in and week out only to see the same persistent figure looking back at you?

The issue may not be what you consume but how much you consume. In reality, portion management is always the most difficult challenge on the road to weight reduction for an individual. If you're looking to reduce, increase, or sustain your weight, maintaining fitness is not only about consuming the right foods but also about having the correct amount of food. This is actually what portion management is: Not eating more (or even less) calories than the body needs. For weight reduction to take effect, one of the very first items discussed in food planning must be portion control.

Portion control is a means of regulating one's consumption by deciding the number of calories in every food serving and restricting intake below a defined level.

The secret to effective weight loss is portion control. Food portion regulation doesn't simply involve having less food, contrary to common opinion, but rather it implies gaining an understanding of how much you consume and the nutrient content of the food. Sticking to one size at a time lets you maintain a balanced nutrient intake from all the various types of foods. Portion control will also help you restrict empty calories while dining out or at a party, making space for healthier options in your day.

In addition to ensuring that you make clean food decisions, portion regulation is often the foundation of a proper diet.

Far too much, without caring about the number of calories we intake, we prefer to eat whatever may be set out on the table in front of us. Loneliness, or intense feelings, such as elation or profound sadness, may contribute to bingeing. It may also result by being confronted with a wide variety of food options. Controlling one's food intake becomes crucial in view of these factors. The emergence of multiple chronic disorders, such as diabetes mellitus, hypertension, excess weight, and unexplained weight loss, may be warded off and managed by sufficient but not unnecessary feeding.

The terms "portion" and "serving" are sometimes used interchangeably by individuals, but servings and portions are not exactly the same amount. And if you are monitoring your calorie consumption and learning food labeling, it counts.

A portion is any quantity of a single food that you chose to place on your plate, while a serving is a prescribed volume of such food based on guidelines on health and diet, such as ChooseMyPlate.gov from the US department of agriculture.

Let's look at an instance here: 1 serving of the cereal and grain category is equivalent to 1 ounce, as per the agriculture department. Not that much. One ounce of white cooked rice is just half a cup or so. The amount of rice you place on your plate might be a lot greater because you may assume you're just consuming one serving of rice while you really consume two or three servings. That's because a half-cup of rice gives your meal about 100 calories, so you may believe you're just consuming 100 calories, but you're really consuming 200 or 300. You will see how the kilocalories will rapidly add up.

Mixing up portions and servings may create confusion, especially when you consume energy-dense foods and high-calorie treats, which can contribute to eating extra calories.

The reference of food portion sizes to ordinary items is a simple way to exercise portion management. For starters, according to the National Institution of Health, a serving of jacket potato is the width of a fist, and one serving of peanut butter is the width of a ping-pong ball.

The more calories you're served, the more you're going to consume, as per the Centers for Disease Control and Prevention. So, turn to smaller dishware as you adapt to consuming smaller servings, which again will render your meals look bigger (and anyway, you feed first with your eyes, right?). This is a minor adjustment that will render the task a little less overwhelming.

Simply equate the serving amounts of items to common objects—instead of having to remember charts of teaspoons, cups, and ounces. A single serving of different foods as compared to regular objects are the following:

- Fruits and vegetables are around the size of your palm.
- Pasta is around the size of a single ice cream scoop.
- Beef, fish, or poultry should be the size of a card deck or the size of your palms (excluding the fingers).
- Snacks such as nachos or pretzels are around the equivalent of cupped nachos.
- A peach is equivalent to the size of a baseball.
- A potato is the equivalent of a mouse of a computer.
- A bagel is compared to the size of a hockey puck.
- A doughnut is compared to the width of a CD.
- Boiled rice should be the width of the wrapping of a cupcake.
- Cheese is the size of your entire thumb (from top to bottom) or the size of a couple of dices.

Shopping List for Lean and Green Diet

Breakfast

- 7 oz. spelt flour
- 1 cup coconut milk
- 1/2 cup alkaline water
- 2 tbsp. grapeseed oil

- 1/2 cup agave
- 1/2 cup blueberries
- 1/4 tsp. sea moss
- 1 cup raspberry
- 1/2 tsp. restrained oil
- 1/2 cup sun-dried tomatoes
- 2 cups spinach
- 1/2 cup coarse cornmeal
- 1/2 tbsp. red pepper
- 1/4 cup baking soda
- 1 1/2 cup all purposes flour, divided
- Kosher salt and freshly ground black pepper
- 1 1/2 oz. can drink beer in style
- 1 code and skin without skin
- 1 cup peeled and spread shrimp, large
- 16 percentiles, shake
- 1 lemon, sliced with cedar wedge
- Tartar sauce, mignon, chimichurri, hot sauce, and malt vinegar, for cedar
- 1 tbsp. ¾ pant
- 1 tbsp. mustard

Mains

- 1 lb. rib eye steak
- 1 tsp. salt
- 1 tsp. cayenne pepper
- ½ tsp. chili flakes
- 3 tbsp. cream
- 1 tsp. olive oil
- 1 tsp. lemongrass
- 1 tbsp. butter

- 1 tsp. garlic powder

Seafood

- ¼ cup chopped fresh cilantro
- ½ cup seeded and finely chopped plum tomato
- 1/3 cup finely chopped red onion
- 10 tbsp. fresh lime juice, divided
- 4–6 oz. boneless, skinless cod fillets
- 5 tbsp. dried unsweetened shredded coconut
- 8 pcs. 6-inch tortillas
- 14 oz. jumbo cooked shrimp, peeled and deveined; chopped
- 4 ½ oz. avocado, diced
- 1 ½ cup tomato, diced
- ¼ cup chopped green onion
- ¼ cup jalapeño with the seeds removed, diced fine
- 1 tsp. olive oil
- 2 tbsp. lime juice
- 1/8 tsp. salt
- 1 tbsp. chopped cilantro

Snacks

- 15 oz. canned white beans, drained and rinsed
- 6 oz. canned artichoke hearts, drained and quartered
- 4 garlic cloves, minced
- 1 tbsp. basil, chopped
- 2 tbsp. olive oil
- Juice of ½ lemon
- Zest of ½ lemon, grated
- Salt and black pepper

Smoothies

- 1 tsp. chia seeds
- ½ cup unsweetened coconut milk
- 1 avocado
- 3/4 frozen burro bananas
- 1 1/2 cups homemade coconut milk
- 1/4 cup walnuts
- 1 tsp. sea moss gel
- 1 tsp. ground ginger
- 1 tsp. soursop leaf powder
- 1 handful kale
- 2 tablespoons extra-virgin olive oil
- 1 onion
- 4 cups fresh baby spinach
- 1 garlic clove, minced
- Zest of 1 orange
- Juice of 1 orange
- 1 cup unsalted vegetable broth
- 2 cups cooked brown rice

Soup and Salad

For the walnuts:

- 2 tbsp. butter
- ¼ cup sugar or honey
- 1 cup walnut pieces
- ½ tsp. kosher salt
- 3 tbsp. extra-virgin olive oil
- ¼ tsp. kosher salt
- 1 head red leaf lettuce, shredded into pieces

- 3 heads endive
- 2 apples
- 1 (8-ounce) camembert wheel

Meat

- 1 lb. beef chuck roast
- 1 fresh lime juice
- 1 garlic clove
- 1 tsp. chili powder
- 2 cups lemon-lime soda
- 1/2 tsp. ssalt
- 2 cups mayonnaise
- 6 plum tomatoes, seeded and finely chopped
- 1/4 cup ketchup
- 1/4 cup lemon juice
- 2 cups seedless red and/or green grapes, halved
- 1 tbsp. Worcestershire sauce
- 2 lb. peeled and deveined cooked large shrimp
- 2 celery ribs, finely chopped
- 3 tbsp. minced fresh tarragon or 3 teaspoon dried tarragon
- salt and 1/4 teaspoon pepper
- 2 cups shredded romaine
- 1/2 cup papaya or peeled chopped mango
- parsley or minced chives

Starches and Grains

- 2 tbsp. extra-virgin olive oil
- 1 onion
- 4 cups fresh baby spinach
- 1 garlic clove, minced

- Zest of 1 orange
- Juice of 1 orange
- 1 cup unsalted vegetable broth
- 2 cups cooked brown rice
- Soup and Salad
- For the walnuts
- 2 tbsp. butter
- ¼ cup sugar or honey
- 1 cup walnut pieces
- ½ tsp. kosher salt
- 3 tbsp. extra-virgin olive oil
- 1 ½ tbsp. champagne vinegar
- 1 ½ tbsp. Dijon mustard
- ¼ tsp. kosher salt
- 1 head red leaf lettuce, shredded into pieces
- 3 heads endive
- 2 apples
- 1 (8-ounce) Camembert wheel

Meal Planner

Meal planning becomes simple in the 5&1 plan when you know the nutritional parameters of a Lean and Green meal according to your lean protein options; a Lean & Green meal contains 5 to 7 ounces of prepared lean protein with three portions of vegetables that are not starchy and up to two portions of healthy fats.

Savor your Lean & Green meal 🍴—Whenever it fits best on your timetable, at any time of day If you're eating out or monitoring your consumption, use the "Lean and Green Meal Nutritional Criteria" given below to direct your choices better:

Nutritional Criteria of L&G

Meal Calories: 250–400 Calories, Meal Carbs ≤ 20 grams of total carbohydrates (ideally < 15 grams), Meal Protein >= 25 grams, Meal Fats 10–20 grams. The three key components of each lean and green meal are Protein, good fats, and carbohydrates. The list of ingredients you would need to make a balanced meal and shop according to your meal schedule is provided below.

Protein is classified into the lean, leaner, and leanest types. Purchase groceries according to recipes of your liking and recipe them to your taste.

Leanest: Pick a 7-oz. (the cooked part, which has 0–4 grams of total fat), then includes 2 healthy fat servings. The leanest options are:

- **Fish:** Cod, haddock, flounder, rough orange, tilapia, grouper, haddock, Mahi Mahi, wild catfish, and tuna (canned in water)
- **Shellfish:** Scallops, crab, lobster, shrimp Game meat: buffalo, deer, elk turkey (ground) or other meat around 98% lean
- **Meatless choices:** 14 egg whites, 2 cups of liquid egg white or liquid egg replacement, 5 oz. of seitan, 1 ½ cups or 2 oz. of 1% cottage cheese, 12 oz. of Non-fat (0%) regular Greek yogurt (approximately 15 g carb per 12 ounces)

Leaner: Pick a 6 oz. (the part cooked), which has 5–9 grams of total fat and includes 1 portion of Healthy Fat.

- **Fish species:** Swordfish, halibut, trout, white meat or Chicken breast skin-free turkey (Ground) or other poultry: 95–97% lean meat
- **Turkey:** Light poultry
- **Meatless choices:** Two entire eggs or four egg whites, two entire eggs and one cup of liquid egg replacer, 1 ½ cups or 12 oz. of 2% cottage cheese, 12 oz. of low-fat (2%) regular Greek yogurt (approximately 15 g carb per 12 oz.)

Lean: Pick a part of 5 oz. Cooked with 10g–20 grams of total fat—no extra portion of healthy fat.

Fish: Tuna (bluefin steak), salmon, catfish farmed, herring, mackerel Lean beef: roasted, ground, steak, lamb pork fillet or porkchop turkey (ground) or other poultry: 85–94% leaner meat.

Turkey or Chicken (Dark Meat)

Meatless choices: 15 oz. extra-firm or firm (bean curd) tofu, 3 whole eggs who (up to 2 days a week), 4 oz. part-skim cheese or reduced-fat (3–6g fat per ounce, 1 cup shredded), and 8 oz. (1 cup) ricotta part-skim cheese (2–3 g of fat per ounce.) 5 oz. tempe.

Healthy Amounts of Fat

There can be around 5 grams of fats and less than 5 grams of carb in a portion of healthy fat. Include 0–2 Healthy Fat Portions daily depending on your options; for Lean: 1 tsp of oil (any sort), 1 tbsp. of normal, low-carb dressing, for the salad 2 tbsp. lowered-fat, low-carb dressing, 5–10 green or black olives 1 ½ ounce. Avocado ⅓ ounce. Simple nuts, such as almonds, pistachios, or peanuts 1 tbsp. of simple seeds, such as sesame, flax, chia, or Seeds of pumpkin ½ tbsp. regular margarine, butter, or mayonnaise.

Green and Lean Meal: The "Greens" make up a substantial proportion of the carbohydrates eaten in the 5&1 diet. Pick three servings from our Green Choices collection for each of Your meals (Lean& Green). We've sorted the choices for vegetables into the amounts of a lower, medium, and higher carb levels. Every one of them is Acceptable on the Optimum Weight 5&1 meal plan; the list assists You to make responsible choices on food. From the Green Choice List, pick 3 servings: 1 serving = ½ cup (except where specified) of vegetables with Around 25 calories and around 5 g of carbohydrates. The Greens include low, moderate, and high carbohydrates.

- **Los carb:** 1 cup endive, green leaf lettuce, Butterhead, romaine, iceberg, collard (fresh/raw), spinach (fresh/raw), mustard greens, watercress, bok choy (raw), spring mix ½ cup: cucumbers, radishes, white mushrooms, sprouts (Mung bean, alfalfa), turnip greens, celery, arugula, escarole, Swiss chard (raw), jalapeño (raw), bok choy (cooked), and nopales.
- **Moderate Carb:** ½ cup: cabbage, eggplant, cauliflower, fennel bulb, asparagus, Mushrooms, Kale, portabella, summer squash (scallop or zucchini) cooked spinach.
- **Higher Carb:** ½ cup: red cabbage, squash, collard, chayote squash(cooked) mustard greens, green or wax beans, broccoli, kabocha squash, (cooked) leeks, Kohlrabi, okra, (any color) peppers, scallions (raw), (crookneck or straightneck) summer squash, Turnips, Tomatoes, Spaghetti Squash, Palm Cores, Jicama, and Swiss (cooked) chard.

Sample Meal Plan Sample

The meal plan of the optimal 5&1 program is very easy and simple to follow. The Fuelings are readily available in pre-packaged and ready to eat from; the only prep you need is for a Lean and Green meal, which is also made easy for you by providing you with the easy recipes and grocery list; a sample meal plan is provided to help you understand the simplicity of this weight loss program. The following are samples of a day on the Optimal 5&1 plan:

- **Sample 1:** Caramel Mocha Shake Fueling
- **Sample 2:** Creamy Double Crisp Peanut Butter Bar Fueling
- **Sample 3:** Roasted Creamy Garlic Smashed Potatoes Fueling
- **Sample 4:** Cinnamon Sugary Sticks Fueling
- **Sample 5:** Chewy Dewy Chocolate Chip Biscuit, Lean and Green meal (your favorite recipe from this book), water intake (check off how many glasses of water you have each day, which should be 8 oz.)

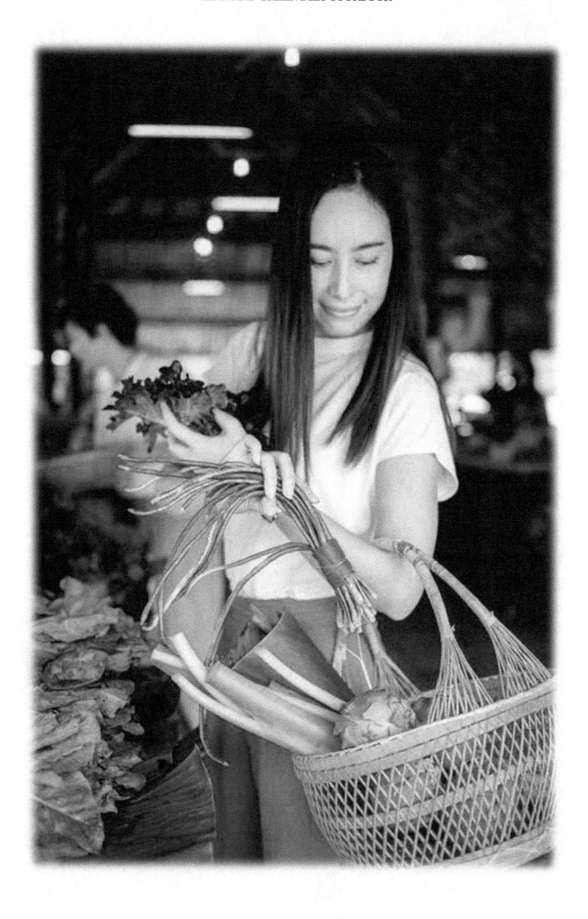

WEIGHT MAINTENANCE

Most "supplies" contain between 100 and 110 calories each, which means you can consume around 1000 calories a day on this diet. As a result of this approach, the "US News" and "World Report" ranked it second on their lists of the best diets for fast weight loss, but 32nd on its list of the best diets for healthy eating. London recognizes that there are other ways to lasting weight loss: "Eat meals and snacks that incorporate lots of products, seeds, nuts, greens, 100% whole grains, eggs, seafood, poultry, greens, low-fat dairy products. Fat, lean meat plus a little indulgence is the best way to lose weight sustainably in the long run." So will the Lean and Green diet help you lose weight?

The amount of weight you lose after following the Lean and Green diet programs depends on factors such as your starting weight as well as your activity and loyalty to following the plan. Lean and Green, launched in 2017, represents a specific lifestyle brand and the coaching community. Previous studies have been done using others products, not the new Lean and Green products. Although the Lean and Green products represent a new line, the company that makes them told US News that they have an identical macronutrient profile, making them interchangeable with the same company's products. Consequently, we believe that the following studies are applicable to the evaluation of this diet. Little specific research has been published on the Lean and Green brand. The studies, like most diets, were small, with numerous dropouts. Research seems to confirm this. On the other hand, the long term expectation is less promising.

A Detailed Look at the Data

According to a 2017 company-sponsored study, more than 70% of overweight adults who received individual behavioral support and underwent this company-supported plan and lost more than 5% of their body weight since their last visit, which is four to 24 weeks.

According to a 2016 study published in the journal Obesity and with partial support from the same company, obese adults lost 8.8% of their body weight after 12 weeks with Lean and Green-style training and products frm this company, and also 12,1% of your bodyweight if you were taking phentermine at the same time, which is a weight-loss drug that can reduce binge eating.

However, the researchers found only one long term study, which indicated no benefit for these 12-month plans. The researchers found that there is also an increased risk of complications such as gallstones on ultra-low-calorie programs.

However, the study found that the effect was reduced beyond six months of reporting the results.

During a small study—designed and funded by this famous company and published in 2010 in the Nutrition Journal, —90 obese adults were randomly assigned to either the low-calorie diet or the 5&1 plan according to government guidelines. People who followed this diet, however, regained more than 4.5 kilograms 24 weeks later, after the calories gradually increased. The others gained only 2 pounds. Compared to the initial exercise, the group that followed this weel-known company's meal plan had more muscle mass and less body fat at week 40, but it did not outperform the control group. Eventually, about half of the well-known company group and more than half of the control group withdrew.

According to a study of 119 overweight or obese type 2 diabetics published in Diabetes Educator in 2008, dieters were randomly assigned to either a diabetes plan or a diet based on the recommendations of the American Association of Diabetes. After 34 weeks, the group of this company had lost an average of 4.5 kilos but regained almost 1.5 kilos after 86 weeks. Over 34 weeks, those who followed the ADA-based diet lost an average of 3 pounds; they got everything back plus an extra pound in 86 weeks. By the end of the year, about 80% had given up.

According to an analysis funded by this company and published in 2008 in the journal Eating and Weight Disorders, researchers analyzed the medical records of 324 people who were on a diet, were overweight or obese, and were also taking a prescribed appetite suppressant. In 12 weeks, they lost an average of 21 pounds; in 24 weeks, they weighed 26 1/2 pounds and 27 pounds in 52 weeks.

Furthermore, for approximately 80% of them, at least 5% of the initial weight had been lost in all three evaluations. This is great if you are obese because losing just 5–10% of your current weight can help prevent some diseases.

However, these numbers are accompanied by some asterisks. First, because they are based on people who completed the 52-week program, they were more likely to lose weight (weight loss was still effective but less pronounced in a cessation analysis).

Second, a review of patient data is given less importance than a study with a control group. Finally, in a survey in which researchers divided dieters into consumer groups, that is, those who recognized that they consume at least two shakes a day at each check-in and those who are inconsistent, it is said the rest; the weight losses of the two groups were not significantly different. The Lean and Green diet has generated headlines throughout the year. Users must enroll in a low-calorie meal plan and then purchase the pre-packaged foods that are part of the chosen plan. In this sitemap, no food group is completely off-limits promising "permanent transformation, one healthy habit at a time."

Although it has many fans, Lean and Green is not cheap. The US News and World Report ranked it second in the rapid weight loss category. In 2018, it was also a popular diet on "Google." The famous "cake chef" Buddy Valastro credits Lean and Green for his recent weight loss.

Do you want to try the Lean and Green diet? Will this really help you lose weight? Here's everything for you: the health implications if they are difficult to follow and the likelihood of reaching your weight loss goal.

How to Maintain Weight

Keeping weight down requires losing weight slowly and steadily, and most of all, being consistent with the Eating Right schedule and workout program. After making some simple changes in eating choices and adding consistent exercise, most of you will lose approximately 3–4 pounds the first week. Then, a weight loss of approximately 1 pound per week can be expected. It is important to do some sort of exercise each day, whether it is weight training, taking a Yoga, Pilates, or Aerobics class, or simply walking. Exercise is critical. Think about this formula:

Eating Right + Exercise

Successful dieters do CHEAT—so plan a cheat day! It means you can choose a day to eat whatever you want at every meal or all day and simply return to your regular healthy eating habits the very next day. Be warned! Cheating on a decadent meal, for example, will make the body rebel. No matter how wonderful the food tastes going down, once the body has adjusted to eating with the proper balance of good healthy food, the shock of those excess calories, fat, and sugar will be difficult to tolerate.

If it is not a cheat day, and the need for something forbidden is felt, treat yourself to a low-fat version or, instead of eating fattening food, purchase a new workout outfit. Looking good and feeling good when you exercise makes it more fun! Learn to treat yourself without using food. Find a special place to alleviate stress. Seek surroundings that are peaceful and beautiful for you. Take time to be pampered.

There is so much pressure on women to look like the women who grace the fashion magazines and are in the endless array of infomercials and television shows. Have you asked yourself—how do they do it? How do they stay slim and fit? It takes more than scheduling workouts at the gym and gulping down a mug of coffee on the way to work. It will not sustain you for very long.

Here are some suggestions for staying slim and healthy at the same time:

Stick to Your Routine: This means, find foods that work for you and will keep you full without increasing your waistline. You have to take the guesswork out of eating your meals, especially breakfast and lunch. It might be scrambled egg whites with vegetables every morning and a grilled chicken salad for lunch—EVERY DAY! You might change the ingredients just a bit by making an omelet instead or substituting salmon for grilled chicken. Develop a routine that makes Eating Right a HABIT rather than a daily BATTLE.

Eat Something Before Going out to a Party: Going out to dinner or to somewhere that is a part of life, and if you eat well during the day, it will allow you a little room when ordering off the menu.

Know What to Do at Parties: All those delicious dishes at parties can pack on the pounds faster than you may think, so make a point of holding a clutch purse in one hand and a glass of wine in another hand—that way, you do not have any hands free to nibble.

Always Take Food with You When You Travel: Do not go anywhere without food. You can always find a piece of fruit, nuts, or a protein bar, so when the cart starts coming down the aisle with nothing but processed foods, it makes it easier just to order water with lemon or tomato juice.

Do Not Allow Yourself to Get Hungry: Before you start feeling those pangs of hunger, take some time to eat ½ of a protein bar, and take your time eating it. It takes a little while for your body to register that it is full and satisfied, so do not rush it!

Exercise: No matter what, find time in your day to exercise. Wake up every morning and figure out when you can exercise by taking a Pilates class or doing Yoga or lifting weights, or getting on the treadmill. MAKE EXERCISE A PRIORITY and NOT AN OPTION. Would you think of going through a day without brushing your teeth or taking a shower? Think about making the time to exercise and find something you enjoy doing and look forward to, even if it is only 20 minutes of Yoga, for example.

Consistency Is the Key: Do whatever it takes to stick with your plan. There are always going to be distractions or issues that arise, so always have a Plan B.

Treat Yourself: If you are going to CHEAT, indulge in foods that are totally worth it. If you really want dessert, the low-fat version doesn't always fit the bill or satisfy the craving. Instead, have a small portion of the 'real' thing. You will find that you appreciate it more when you have it in moderation.

Tips for Weight Maintenance

Here are a few of the tips you can use to practice controlling your portions to lose weight:

Measure Portions to Avoid Overeating

Portion regulation helps with an appreciation of serving quantities through consuming only the proper quantity of every food. As a guide, use the "Nutrition Facts" table used on all pre-prepared items. The serving size, accompanied by the number of servings contained in the package, is the first entry. Much of the details below depend on the quantity of food in a single serving, like carbohydrates, fats, and sodium. If you consume double the serving size, you have double the amount of calories, carbohydrates, and fats mentioned. Measure the snack or count the number of cookies where possible, for instance, and be sure you don't consume further than you planned.

You have to weigh them in order to understand the exact portions of food. Measuring containers and bowls can aid, but overfilling a cup or bowl can be simple. Using a modern food scale, the most effective way to calculate meals is by weight.

Serve Your Food on a Plate

Placing the meals on a plate instead of consuming out of the tub, jar, or served dish is another perfect way to maintain portion sizes. Fill half of your dish with lettuce and vegetables for dinner and lunch, and then split the other half into proteins and carbohydrates. If you have to look for a second portion, you can overeat less frequently.

Limit Nibbling on Food while You're Preparing it

You ought to give up grazing in order to consume fewer. It's enticing to taste the food while you're preparing it, but it's best to wait before the dinner is made. By the same point, it's tempting to neglect to count calories that were not on your own plate, so avoid taking leftovers from the plate of your kid or partner. You will broaden your mind to the excess calories you gain in a day by maintaining a food journal. For a few days, write down any bite you take or drink you sip, and then read the list. The findings may shock you and promote better dietary behaviors.

Don't Bring Extra Food onto The Table

Set aside any food that won't be placed on your plate once you settle down to eat. If you had to pull the food out once again, you would be less motivated for a further serving. Even overeating may be induced by only having food lying inside arms reach. Concealing leftover food, quick snacks, and sweets somewhere you can't see them all the time will help you consume little.

Split the Food

Owing to the large serving sizes that restaurants offer, dining out is a significant contributor to bingeing. Try consuming just half the food the next time you head out. You'll conserve half the amount of calories. By packing up some extra portion of "to go" before you even feed, you may ask your waiter to help. Dividing a meal with a mate is yet another simple and inexpensive way to consume less.

Include More Veggies

If you are going to overeat something, the safest way is to eat vegetables. Next, load your bowl with veggies with a minimum of five servings a day. Veggies are easier to afford and very low in fat and calories, but high in fiber as well as other phytonutrients and phytonutrients. That's very effective in helping you preserve good fitness. When it comes to loading the plate, nutritionists advocate concentrating on non-starchy vegetables.

Consume as much Caesar salad as you want to spice up the meal (such as kale, broccoli, tomato, celery, and zucchini). Include herbs for flavor, but retain the prescribed portion size with fats, protein, and carbohydrates. A perfect way to fuel up without eating more calories is to incorporate more veggies into your recipes. Begin your dinner with lettuce, finish your lunch with vegetables and carrots, and add your morning eggs to your preferred steamed veggies.

Use Plates That Are Smaller

Over the decades, when plate dimensions have risen, so have food portions. To hold portions in control, pick 9-inch plates for grownups and 7-inch plates for kids. Your plate will appear fuller; your subconscious will be fooled into believing that you have more fuel.

Always Listen to Your Body

We're all guilty of multitasking. Try to stop feeding when watching TV or while you're on the phone. Studies suggest that mindless consumption contributes to excess weight, so make sure to calculate the right portion sizes and actually consume your treats from a bowl.

It sounds so easy, but in reality, many of us let our minds rule our bodies rather than the other way around, particularly when it comes to emotional eating. Ask yourself whether you're very hungry before getting a snack or whether you're listening to your desires or feeding out of habit. Consume less by not using eating to cope or distract you; instead, take a stroll. And don't just grab a bag of snacks while you're watching a movie or buy popcorn while you're at the cinema.

Be Smart About Salads

Thought food portions for salads wouldn't count? Often remember, it's good to be aware of your chopped vegetables and portions as much as for other meals. For optimum eating and a healthy mix of ingredients, figure out how to make the best of your next salad.

Drink Water Before Eating

Do not forget to consume a ton of water prior to eating before you get to sort your meals. One of the easiest strategies is to drink a glass of water half an hour before a meal or whatever you snack. This is because you're more apt to consume extra while you're dehydrated. It ensures you get more water throughout from getting a huge glass of water, but you're still less likely to get that large of a portion amount.

Use a Plate or Your Palm as a Guide

Use the plate or palm guideline to get a sense of the quantity of starch, calories, fats, and vegetables to have in a serving. Divide the portion into half a dish of low-starch vegetables, a fifth of a plate of protein, a fourth of a plate of complex carbohydrates, and half a tablespoon of fat. Use the palm to 'measure' out reasonable quantities, and use it in combination with the plate principle.

Note to maintain the size of your hand's palm for protein, your finger's tip as a butter serving size, a fourth of an avocado per serving, and no more than the width of a matchbox to measure cheese.

Use the Same Plates and Bowls

Think about it: when it's placed on a large plate, a regular pasta serving seems even smaller, implying that after eating, we're more inclined to feel dissatisfied. Whether the plate is rather big or tiny, or whether the bowls are wider than you've had before, it's very simple to get a bit confused in your mind. You assume you have the same quantity; however, you're having more because of the illusion of the portion.

Change Your Spoon Size

Admit it; you eat more than soup with your oversized spoons. Okay, it's time to quit the trend because evidence suggests that we consume fewer if we use a teaspoon instead of a tablespoon, according to experts. So, if possible, pick a smaller scooper, specifically when it comes to calorie-rich snacks like ice cream.

Another Pro Tip: Consider switching the broad serving spoons too; it's tougher to put on huge quantities with a smaller version.

Eat Slowly and Savor

Eating quickly makes you more apt to skip the hunger and fullness indicators. Taking your time with a meal, actually treasuring each taste, encourages you to experience the meal further and can ensure that you don't overeat what you're consuming. This implies not pacing in front of the TV, over the countertop, or gulping down the dinner. Sit and eat mindfully and frequently. Eating quickly and in a rush, food will feel less enjoyable.

Mind to ensure your foods are balanced in terms of macro and micronutrients, a source of nutrition, good fats, and complex carbs to make these portion-controlled meals more fulfilling. Have low GI (gastrointestinal) effects with carbohydrates, such as lentils, chickpeas, beans, brown rice, quinoa, and butternut squash. They're all excellent energy sources you absorb slowly and offer you energy for a long period. Include healthier fats, such as avocado, almonds, nuts, and olive oil because the fat makes us remain fuller, plus it's very nice for your skin, hair, and body. And, of course, high-quality poultry, such as meat, sustainably captured salmon, and leaner varieties of grass-fed beef and lamb if necessary. This aims to enhance the quality of the fatty acids found in the meat. Add more legumes, tofu, and kimchi for vegetarian forms of protein. Not only is stuff like lentils (chickpeas, lentils) a decent supply of carbs, they add up and are also a very nice source of protein.

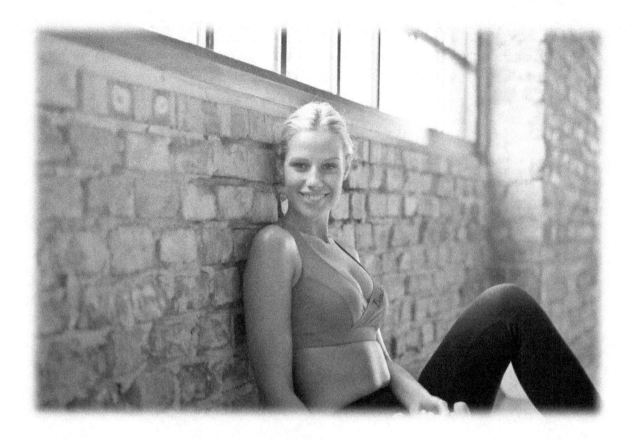

CONCLUSION

The logic behind the Lean and Green diet is that eating healthy recipes will make you feel full for a long time (not similarly to foods that are high in carbohydrates and saturated fat). That's why it focuses on increasing the consumption of whole foods and reducing dependence on fast commercial foods and other unhealthy foods.

The program has earned worldwide acclaim for its ability to deliver sustainable results without complicating the meal program for people. It places very few restrictions on food and inspires people to choose a healthier version of their daily food without compromising taste or nutrition.

Choosing the right diet or program had also become difficult as the industry flourished. Many diets claim to have specific health problems while helping a diet lose weight.

Unlike other diets, the Lean and Green diet is not designed for a specific health condition. It is designed according to the dieters' needs to achieve the ideal weight and the healthy lifestyle you want.

When you desire a structure and need to lose weight rapidly, the Lean and Green diet is the perfect solution.

The extremely low-calorie eating plans of the Lean and Green diet will definitely help you shed more pounds.

Before you start any meal replacement diet plan, carefully consider if it is truly possible for you to continue with a specific diet plan. When you have decided to stick with Lean and Green and make progress with your weight loss goal, ensure you have a brilliant knowledge about optimal health management to enable, and archive desired results effortlessly in the shortest time period.

The Lean and Green diet program is a stress-free and easy-to-follow program. It is a cool way to start a journey to your health.

Thank you!

LEAN AND GREEN DIET FOR WEIGHT LOSS

The Ultimate and Easy Solution to Lose Weight in Critical Points Without Counting Calories. How to Boost Your Metabolism, Increase Energy, And Shape Your Body

© Copyright 2021 - All rights reserved.

Table of Contents

INTRODUCTION

Experts say that the Lean and Green diet can help you because it is essentially less caloric when it comes to weight loss.

If you are interested in trying this, consider working with an experienced registered dietitian, who can help you stay adequately fed as you strive to achieve your desired weight.

The most desirable weight plan, to begin with, is Initial Plan 5&1: eat 5 foods per day, plus a low-carb lean meal and a low-carb elective snack.

Although Initial Plan 5&1 is reasonably restrictive, Protection Segment 3 & 3 allows for a greater variety of less processed foods and snacks, which can also make weight loss easier, and more persistent for a long period.

The bottom line is that the Lean and Green weight loss plan promotes weight loss via low-calories pre-packaged meals, low-carb homemade food, and personalized coaching.

Lean and Green diet enhances weight loss through branded products known as fueling, while the homemade **entrées** are referred to as the lean and green meals. Fuelings are specifically made up of over 60 low-carb items but are high in probiotic cultures and proteins. They ultimately contain friendly bacteria that can help to boost gut health and include: cookies, bars, puddings, shakes, soups, cereals, and pasta.

Looking at the listed foods, you might think they are relatively high in carbs, which is understandable, but the fuelings are composed so that they are lower in sugar and carbs than the traditional versions of similar foods. It is possible by using small portions and sugar substitutes. Many of the fuelings are packed with isolated soy protein and whey protein powder. Those interested in the Lean and Green diet plan but not interested or without chances to cook are provided with pre-made low-carb meals. These meals are referred to as Flavors of Home and can sufficiently replace the lean and green meals.

The Lean and Green diet is an idea of a well-known company. It comprises pre-purchased portioned snacks and meals, low-carb lean and green (homemade) meals, and continuous coaching based on facilitating fat and weight loss.

The promoting company explicitly states that by working with its team of coaches and following the Lean and Green diet as required, you will achieve a "lifelong transformation, one healthy habit at a time."

Therefore, to be successful with this diet plan, you should stick to the fuelings supplemented by veggie, meat, and healthy fat **entrée** daily; as a result, you will be nourished and satisfied. Although you will be consuming low calories, you will not be losing a lot of muscle since you will be feeding on lots of fiber, protein, and other vital nutrients. Your calories, as an adult, will not exceed 800–1,000. You can lose 12 pounds in 12 weeks if you follow the optimal weight 5&1 plan option.

Since you will curb your carb intake on this diet plan, you will naturally shed fat because the carb is the primary source of energy; therefore, if it is not available, the body finds a fat alternative, which implies that the body will be forced to break down your fats for energy and keep burning fat.

I gladly welcome you to try out the Lean and Green diet. If strictly followed, you can be sure that the results will be waiting for you at the end of the program. As you already know, recipes for the Lean and Green diet are rich in nutrients and are designed to help you eliminate unwanted weight, but in the long run, you'll need to use the recipes to develop a smarter eating habit. For long-term results that transcend the Lean and Green program's duration, you should strive to live on a diet filled with lots of fruits, whole grains, lower carbs, and vegetables. As you explore the rich recipes in this book, feel free to make more research and add a bit of spice to the guide if you feel up to it. However, be sure to cross-check your experimentation with an expert on the diet, with your Lean and Green program coach, or feedback with us.

Cheers!

WHAT IS YOUR IDEAL WEIGHT?

The Optimal Weight 5&1 Strategy, which requires five fuels a day, is adopted by most dieters. You may select from more than 60 choices, including shakes, soups, bars, biscuits, and pudding, many of which contain a probiotic that the company claims encourage digestive health and high-quality protein. Your sixth regular meal, which you may take in at any point, is made up of prepared lean protein, three portions of veggies, and good fats.

You'll collaborate with Lean and Green coaches while on a diet, and further, become a group member to support your progress. You'll collaborate with Lean and Green coaches while on a diet, and further, become a group member to support your progress. When you hit your target weight, it is potentially simpler to move from the diet, and your old habits are substituted with new ones. Via its Optimum Fitness 3&3 Plan, the company delivers a specific range of items tailored for weight management.

For people searching for a more customizable yet higher-calorie diet, Lean and Green also provides the Ideal Weight 4&2&1 Package, which involves four fuelings, two lean and green meals, and one healthy snack, such as a fruit or a sweet potato portion. The company also promotes special programs for people with asthma, nursing mothers, individuals with gout, the elderly, and teenagers.

Lean and Green Diet eating strategies somewhat differ based on how much weight you need to lose and how early you are in the path of weight reduction, although all diets consist of two key elements: lean and green meals and fueling.

Fuelings are Lean and Green's pre-packaged meals intended to be "nutritively interchangeable food replacements that are carb-controlled and low-fat," with choices varying from bars, cookies, and shakes to more nutritious meals, such as Spinach Mac & Cheese with pesto cooked by your own, lean and green meals, and rely on lean protein, balanced fats, and vegetables that are from lower-carb. Plans differ depending on the amount of regular recommended lean and green meals and fueling (see below) that steadily growing in calories and carbohydrates.

- **5&1 Schedule:** 1 lean and green meal, and 5 fuelings from 800 to 1,000 calories.

- **4&2&1 Schedule**: 2 lean and green meals, 5 fuelings, and 1 nutritious snack from 1,100 to 1,300 calories.

- **5&2&1 Schedule:** 2 lean and green meals, 5 fuelings, and 2 nutritious snacks from 1,300 to 1,500 calories.

- **3&3 Schedule:** 3 lean and green meals and fuelings from 1,500 to 1,800 calories, and one fruit or low-fat dairy serving is deemed a nutritious snack.

To encourage weight reduction, Lean and Green depends on intensively reducing calories. Most fuelings produce about 100-110 calories, which ensures you can eat about 1,000 calories per day on this diet.

What Is the Perfect Target of People?

The simplicity of meal replacement programs that take the guessing out of weight management has long attracted customers. That's why the successful meal replacement program in Lean and Green Diet is suggested for individuals who are too busy to prepare all three meals daily; it also reduces the hassle of shopping for every item by offering a range of food options in fuelings and supplying them to doorsteps. The Lean and Green Diet is essentially intended to shed more than 15 lbs. of weight for healthier adults. However, they still provide programs customized to fit with those who have specific fitness or lifestyle conditions. Lean and Green provides suggestions for adults over 65 and inactive, relatively active individuals, people who have little weight to lose, persons who choose to add more carbs into their diet, and plans for people with gout. It specifies that it should be practiced with a specialist's guidance for diabetes type 1 or type 2. Also, for those aged from 13 to 18 years, it provides a teenage package, making it one of the relatively few consumer diets accessible for teenagers.

What Are the Benefits

There are additional benefits to the Lean and Green diet that can improve weight reduction and general health.

Simple to Adopt

The diet depends primarily on pre-packaged foods; on the 5&1 program, you are only liable for cooking one meal a day.

What is more, to make things easy to execute, each schedule comes with food logs and a sample diet plan.

Although you are expected to prepare 1 to 3 lean and green meals every day, they are quick to create depending on the diet since the package provides unique recipes and a selection of food choices.

Besides, to supplement lean and green foods, many that are not involved in cooking may purchase prepared meals labeled Flavors of Home.

Blood Pressure Can Improve

Via weight loss and restricted sodium intake, lean and Green programs can help improve blood pressure. Although the Lean and Green diet has not been explicitly studied, a 40-week report showed a substantial decrease in blood pressure in 90 people with excess weight and obesity on a modified regimen.

Also, all lean and Green nutrition plans are designed to have less than 2,300 mg of sodium a day, but it is upon you to select low sodium lean and green meal alternatives.

Numerous health associations recommend consuming fewer than 2,300 mg of sodium a day, including the College of Medicine, the American medical association, and the U.S. Department of Agriculture (USDA). This is because high salt consumption is correlated with an elevated likelihood of high blood pressure and heart failure in salt-sensitive people.

Offers Continuing Assistance

Lean and Green health trainers are accessible for weight reduction and maintenance services throughout their programs.

As mentioned above, one research found a substantial association between the quantity of Lean and Green 5&1 Plan coaching sessions and increased weight loss.

Besides, literature shows that long-term weight management can be helped by obtaining a health coach or psychologist.

Lean and Green Diet Effective

Caloric restriction is essential for weight loss, and with an 800–1,000 calories dietary schedule, the 5&1 program is particularly conducive to fast shedding pounds. With the right amount of protein per serving, carbohydrates are also kept minimal, which is perfect for successful weight loss in most cases.

Besides carb and calorie restrictions, many health benefits, including increased glucose processing, body structure improvements, decreased risk of cardiovascular risk factors, and other risk factors for diseases.

But the 5&1 may not be for everyone as it can be hazardous for health to lose weight too fast and extreme calorie restriction, and you will certainly not feel healthy, though muscle loss is also a possibility. 800–1,000 calories, in general, is very poor.

However, if not applied for extended periods, eating 800-1,000 calories can be healthy and efficient for weight loss.

Research shows that too few calories will influence your metabolism over time, leading you to regain weight loss.

But this may also be attributed to long-term habits because when it comes to the discrepancies between people, there are also several different factors to consider. Weight loss is not always easy, and it can be much more challenging to keep it off, but permanent lifestyle changes are needed.

Lean and Green also suggests exercising 30 minutes daily, which is also vital for maintaining weight and good health.

Research suggests that it's crucial to set sensible goals based on a character's needs, preferences, and contemporary health. Diets ought to be nutritionally ok for every man or woman, which once more may additionally vary.

However, the scientific literature does, in reality, support using meal replacements as a powerful option for weight reduction and sort 2 diabetes. One study that takes a look at 119 individuals found that element-controlled meal replacements yielded considerably more weight reduction and upkeep of the load than a general, self-decided on meals-primarily based weight loss program after 12 months.

There was also a study that compared the Lean and Green 5&1 weight loss program plus phone aid (OPT) to one decreased-calories 4&2&1 self-guided plan, and also to a self-directed decreased-calories manage food plan. A group of 198 individuals was randomly assigned to these eating regimens for evaluation at some point of 16 weeks.

The OPT's and MED's individuals experienced considerably more weight reduction and belly fats than the self-directed control weight-loss plan group. And the study concluded that the considerable weight reduction difference was correlated with the meal replacements and make contact with aid.

Keep in mind, even though the study was funded by a private company, yet other numerous studies observed that education is very useful for weight loss.

Is it sustainable and healthful for a long time, appropriately? There isn't sufficient proof to make that judgment.

However, the pre-packaged meals from Lean and Green are processed to a degree. Hence, there are positive delivered elements along with meal components, but also processed oils that might not be healthful in huge quantities. Nevertheless, Lean and Green is a clean label product, so there are not any synthetic colorations, flavors, or sweeteners

But it's best cautioned to get regular checkups and preferably not continue to be on a program for too long after you've reached your loss-weight goal. Although they propose their 3&3 plan when you've reached your goal, it's in the long run that the man or woman decides whether or not they need to hold with an application and training.

Also, U.S. News and World Report rank Lean and Green #2 for excellent weight reduction diets, #10 for nice industrial food plan plans, although it ranks #27 for wholesome diets.

So, once more, it could be a unique weight loss program, although for health could not be worth sustaining it in the long haul.

This is where Lean and Green claims to stand out among different diet programs. The training patently helps maintain the clients' advantages, influencing them, leading to extra consistency.

Their manual is also very beneficial as it offers you all the fundamentals to effortlessly check with it at any time. Lean and Green also gives meal pointers and recipes via multiple social structures.

How Does Lean and Green Assist You with Getting You Fit?

Lean and Green depends on strongly confining calories to advance weight reduction. Most fuelings drift around 100–110 calories each, which means you could take in about 1,000 calories for every day on this diet. Because of Lean and Green's sensational methodology, U.S. News and World Report positioned it #2 in its rundown of Best Fast Weight-Loss Diets, however, #32 in its rundown of Best Diets for Healthy Eating. "Present moment, it appears to be inconceivable not to shed probably a few pounds; you're eating a large portion of the calories most grown-ups expand," it said. "The drawn-out standpoint is less encouraging."

London concurs that there's a particular way to deal with enduring weight reduction: "'Eating dinners and tidbits that join heaps of produce, 100% entire grains, nuts, seeds, vegetables, low-fat dairy items, eggs, poultry, fish, and lean hamburger in addition to certain extravagances is the most ideal approach to get more fit economically for the long stretch."

Lean and Green is a fast weight reduction or maintenance method that prescribes a combination of bought, refined foods labeled fueling and lean and green home-made meals. There's no carbohydrates or calories counting. Instead, as part of six-or-so small meals every day, members apply water to a powdered meal or unwrap a cookie.

The purpose of introducing fueling is to curb the cravings and a nutritiously balanced meal to keep the dieter satiated.

The highly nutritious and low-calorie nature of most foods you'll eat on the Lean and Green diet as fueling provides various flavors for different taste buds, which curbs any sort of sweet or savory cravings without compromising your plan.

Intake of fresh, whole foods such as meat, fruits, and vegetables are adequately administered in lean and green meals, keeping your diet healthy and balanced.

Although Lean and Green's 5&1 plan with the 800 to 1,000 calories count per day is intended for optimal weight loss, there are also other plans with higher calorie intake to suit everyone's nutritional needs.

Achieving Amazing Results for Your Ideal Weight

If you're struggling with your program and wondering how you can be successful, there are a few things that you need to do. Our body has to adjust to new eating plans and exercise, and you may struggle a bit to reach your goals. This is normal and it shouldn't hold you back. Here's how you can ensure that you're successful.

Work at It Each Day

You should be prepared each day to do what it takes to get in shape. You should have meal plans ready to go, and you should be ready to get in some sort of activity, even if it's just 15 minutes. The more you prepare for getting in shape each day, the better off you're going to be. Make sure you write things down and use gadgets to track calories, the number of steps you have taken, etc. This should be a part of your daily routine by the end of your first week.

Don't Quit

You can't quit when you have just begun. Once you lay down the foundation, you'll see just how easy the process starts to be. You'll begin to feel better because you're eating well, you'll have fewer cravings for bad foods, and you will be getting stronger because you're beginning to exercise more often. Don't sabotage yourself by quitting; you have to keep going.

Don't Allow Failure to Win

If you fail and don't do what is required one day or eat foods that you shouldn't eat, you can't allow this to sabotage you. It's okay to fail because we have all done it when it comes to diet and exercise. All you do is pick yourself up again and get back on track. Your new lifestyle isn't gone for good because you ate cheesecake the night before. Every so often, you should indulge a bit because we are all human. If you stick to a 90% healthy lifestyle and only indulge every so often, you're still going to do fine.

It's in the Mind

Getting in shape is very much a mental process, so once you overcome this fact, there's no limit on what you can achieve. We all have it inside of ourselves to get into shape, and you're one of these people. A positive attitude goes a long way towards your success, and once you are positive, you'll see the results start to show up. The best thing you can do is to start now. Once you make this commitment, there's nothing that will stand in your way. A healthy lifestyle and a good body are easier to achieve than you realize; it's there waiting for you, so go out and make it happen now.

Change It Up

You want to vary the routine that you do. If you perform the same routine, your body will get used to it over time. You should have several routines you can alternate with. This will force the body to work hard, and in turn, you'll burn more calories with each exercise session. You should also introduce new exercises from time to time to challenge the muscles in new ways. This will increase the amount of fat you burn even more. The muscles need a good challenge to keep growing, and you'll break through those plateaus that can hold you back.

Don't Forget a Rest Day

Intervals work well, but you should have at least one full rest day. The entire body needs to recover from intense exercise so make sure you have one rest day during the week. You can also alternate exercises, so you don't work for the same muscle groups. For example, you could do all chest intervals one day and all leg intervals the next day with some cardio thrown in that routine.

The Power of "a Plan"

When people have no plan, they will simply be **drifting.** Daily circumstances will push them one way one day and another direction the next. Life just "happens" to them.

But YOU have a plan. Your exercise and nutrition plan is the one in this book.

Every month you will be using this plan to *master more skills* for being fit.

How you go about doing those things is determined by your mindset and motivation.

It is easy to make plans and then ignore them. That is what a lot of people do.

You must assert that you are in control of what goes on in your life. To get back in shape, you must assert control over your exercise and nutrition.

The Power of Persistence

Being persistent is an overwhelming factor for success in virtually any endeavor. It is the only way you will find out how successful you can be at any given undertaking.

Talent and other innate gifts do play some role in how good you eventually become. The most important thing is to understand that you will only realize your full potential by working persistently on a task. In this course, you have no idea how successful you can be until you do the work! This program is about realizing your unique potential. Understand that at the start, you have no idea how successful you can be. Embrace the growth mindset. In the real world, you never really know what you can do until you work at it!

Positive Energy

Taking on a new challenge will require the best effort you can muster. One of the most important conditions for putting out your best effort will be lots of positive energy.

The energy will come from yourself and your attitude, and those around you.

You begin every day with a "can-do" attitude and get excited about your training and what you will accomplish. You feel the power of your enthusiasm propelling you to make changes and do the things you know are needed.

Positive energy is contagious. When you dive into a task with positive enthusiasm, it energizes those around you to feel good and do their best.

Positive energy will lift you and move you ahead. Negative energy will do just the opposite.

Negative energy feels like it sucks the air out of a room. Tasks that may have seemed a little difficult now become impossible.

Having a positive attitude can make that hard work seems enjoyable. It helps you surge forward and embrace the next challenge.

A negative attitude can do just the opposite. It can stop you in your tracks before you even get started. Negativity hangs in the air like a bad smell and can undercut everything you try to do.

Being around negative people can drain your energy quickly. For them, life appears to be a trudge from one bad experience to another. They find faults in everything. They will assure you that trying to get back in good condition is going to fail.

You should stay as far away from these people as possible. They will do nothing but suck the energy out of you. They are the last people you want to be around when you are trying to do something difficult.

Hang out with positive and enthusiastic people, particularly about your desire to get back in good condition. Their positive energy will multiply your energy.

Take Action

If someone delays acting, the chances are that they won't do anything. Procrastination becomes a normal way of life.

Many have good intentions. But they avoid **acting.** The longer they put off taking action, the less likely it is that they will ever DO something.

High Achievement

Being a high achiever means that you may routinely place a lot of extreme expectations on yourself. It is likely that "doing a great job" is one way you got a lot of your approval and recognition in your life. This approval may have come from parents, family, co-workers, **etc.** In short, you were "proving yourself."

It is possible that you are being driven may still be a means of trying to prove yourself. If you recognize this and drop the emotional overhead, you will probably do just as good a job but feel some satisfaction in your accomplishment.

Discipline

You are **committed** to getting back in shape. How do you get yourself to **do** what is necessary, particularly when you may not **want** to do something at a specific time?

The word discipline comes to mind. This means doing something you know you **should,** even though your body may not **want to.** The **real** successes in life come from having the discipline to do something that may not be appealing at first.

You have exercised discipline in your life before, probably many times. If you built a successful career, the early work was not easy and often not fun. If you mastered a difficult subject in school, you probably had to endure many hours of difficult study. If you learned to play a musical instrument, you had to do a lot of practice when you were a real novice.

The good news is that the longer you stick with an exercise program, the more it becomes enjoyable!

Resources and Products

Together with providing meal replacements, Lean and Green also offers resources that showcase the best methods to prepare your lean and green meals.

Though the diet plan does not require specific recipes, broiling, grilling, poaching, and baking are the recommended methods for cooking meats and other options of proteins.

You can utilize Lean and Green's Pin interest board of plan-compliant recipes if you need fresh meal ideas.

Another resource that makes the Lean and Green program unique is the availability of a member who successfully finished the program. This person, usually referred to as a coach, is there to cheer you on as you embark on your weight-loss journey.

Modifications

There is not much room for improvement in the Lean and Green diet plan because it depends wholly on strict calorie-controlled prepared meals and proprietary meal replacement products.

Calories are limited to as low as 800–1,000 each day in the 5&1 plan. As a result, it is not suitable for people who engage in rigorous exercises and pregnant women.

Do note that extreme calorie restrictions can result in menstrual changes, fatigue, headaches, or brain fogs, due to that. You should not use the 5&1 option on a long-term basis.

Numbers of Calories You Should Eat on the Lean and Green Diet

Since every person is specific (E.G., Weight, age, interest levels), caloric needs couldn't be the same for anybody trying to preserve a healthy weight. For instance, a 200 lb. man can have different caloric needs than a 130 lb. lady.

So, with the 3&3 plan, energy variety goes from 1,200–2,500 calories per day.

Now with the Optimal Weight 5&1 Plan, calories variety goes from 800–1,000 in keeping with day, even as the Optimal Weight 4&2&1 plan tiers from 1,100–1,300 energy in keeping with day. Both of those meal plans are designed to supply a healthy quantity of nutrients for each man and woman.

And even though the 5&1 plan has fewer calories typical, it elicits a fats-burning conducive to the usage of fats shops for power.

But the plan which is excellently suitable for you'll be determined beforehand when you buy a program and seek advice from a coach, who will help you during the program's duration.

Exercises to Accelerate the Weight-Loss Process

Working the Upper Body

Including the upper body, body-weight strength training is an important part of a lifestyle change to improve your figure and health. A majority of recommended exercises tend to be focused on the lower body and ignore the upper half, which will decrease the effectiveness of your workouts and results. Adding upper body exercises to your body-weight training program should occur at least twice per week with a minimum of one pushing and one pulling movement. This form of exercise can add important muscle that can help burn fat twenty-four hours a day and improve the chest, back, shoulders, and arms. The movement will become easier, leaving you stronger and able to perform the activities that you love. It's time to reverse the effects of aging and reclaim your body with body-weight strength training.

Exercises can be performed in supersets, groups of three exercises, or a full circuit:

Push Up

Muscles: Pectorals, triceps, deltoids, core.

Reps: 8

- Begin with the hands directly under the shoulders with the elbows extended, torso fully extended, and the feet together with toes tucked under them.

- The body is in a straight line with the butt, thighs, and abs held tight.

- Slowly lower the body to the floor, keeping the elbows close to the body.

- Once almost touching the floor, push into the ground to move the body back into the starting position.

- **Regression:** perform on the knees or spread the feet to shoulder width.

- **Progression:** perform with only one leg on the ground.

Superman

Muscles: Middle and lower back, lats, abs, obliques.

Sets: 3 **Reps:** Count of 3

- Lie facing down with arms fully extended the head and legs stretched behind you.

- Lift your chest and your arms and your legs off of the floor by curving your back. Only the tops of your quads and your lower abdomen should be in contact with the floor.

- Embrace for a tally of three while clutching your abdomen and oblique.

- Return to the starting position for a count of one and repeat.

- **Regression:** hold arms along the side of your body and raise as you raise your legs.

- **Progression:** hold arms at 90-degree angles to your body and raise as you raise your legs.

Shoulder Walk Out

Muscles: Traps, pectorals, triceps, deltoids, core.

Sets: 1, **Reps:** 3

- Begin by standing with feet together, and hips bent to place the hands on the ground as close to the feet as possible.

- Squeeze the butt, thighs, and abs to maintain a flat back throughout the exercise.

- Walk hands forward in three to four inches increments while keeping the feet in place until in the push-up starting position.

- Walk hands backward in three to four inches increments, returning to the bent over starting position.

- **Regression:** perform on the knees, beginning with hands in front of the knees.

- **Progression:** walk hands past the push-up position to extend the body as far as possible without allowing the hips to drop or the back to round.

Mountain Climbers

Muscles: Quadriceps, chest, glutes, hamstrings, shoulders

Sets: 3 **Reps:** 30 seconds

- Begin in a push-up position.

- Starting with one of your legs, flex your knee and hip simultaneously to carry your knee up and under your hip and your foot on the floor. Your other leg must continue fully extended.

- Jump to inverse your legs' site by spreading the bent leg and concurrently bending the straight leg until it is up and under the hip.

- Carry on alternating in this fashion for the prescribed total time, rest for 30 seconds, and continue.

- Regression: instead of jumping, step the knee up under the hip placing your foot on the floor, and step back into the push-up position. Continue with the other knee.

- Progression: instead of resting for 30 seconds, use that time to do push-ups.

Hip Raiser

Muscles: Triceps, shoulders, glutes, hamstrings.

Sets: 3 **Reps:** 8

- Sit on the floor with your back straight and legs together, extended straight in front of you.

- Place arms by your sides and hands flat on the ground facing forward.

- Raise your hips, keeping your arms straight and feet flat on the floor with knees bent at a 90-degree angle. Your body will be in a straight line from the knees up. Squeeze the glutes.

- Hold this position for a count of three and slowly return to the starting position.

- Regression: lift the hips only halfway.

- Progression: once the pelvis is raised, lift one leg parallel to the floor, hold for a count of 3, and return to the starting position.

Working the Lower Body

The muscles of our hips and thighs from the base of support for the body. These muscles allow us to rise and keep us upright when we stand and move our legs to walk, run, jump, land, and change direction. The lower body is the foundation of balance, and without the proper functioning of this state, our mobility is greatly decreased. Keeping these muscles in optimal working condition is essential in maintaining our quality of life and independence as we age.

Lower body body-weight training also has positive influences on your overall health and well-being. Disease prevention, improved movement, and emotional and psychological advancements are all benefits of regular physical activity and will aid in everyday living now and in the future.

Exercises can be performed in supersets, groups of three exercises, or a full circuit.

Hip Press

Muscles: Glutes, hamstrings, lower back.

Sets: 3 **Reps:** 8

- Lie on your back with your knees bent so that your feet are flat on the floor.

- Push through the heels to raise the hips.

- Pause at the top of the movement before returning to the starting position.

- Keep the butt, thighs, and abs tight throughout the movement.

- Do not hyperextend the lower back; maintain a straight line from knees to shoulders at all times.

- Regression: do not fully extend the hips, only raise halfway up.

- Progression: perform the exercise with one leg by grabbing the other leg with the hands and pulling the knee to the chest.

Single Leg Glute Bridge

Muscles: Glutes, hamstrings, quadriceps.

Sets: 3 **Reps:** 8

- Lie on your back with your knees bent so that your feet are flat on the floor.

- Raise one leg off the floor and extend it straight out.

- Depress via your heel on the floor and thrust hips up, raising the gluteals off of the mat. Carry on until the hips are parallel with your upper body (torso). Hold for a count of 3.

- Lower your hips to the floor.

- Complete all the repetitions for one set before changing legs.

- Regression: switch legs after every repetition.

- Progression: execute the repetitions at a fast pace without holding the position.

Side Lunge

Muscles: Quadriceps, glutes, hamstrings.

Sets: 3 **Reps:** 8

- Begin in a standing position with feet together and hands on hips or waist.

- Keep your left leg straight, step out to the side with your right leg bending at the knee.

- Push off the right leg and return to the start position.

- Regression: instead of pushing back up to the starting position, stay low and slide across to the other side.

- Progression: reach for your right foot with your left hand and vice versa on the opposite side.

Single Leg Deadlift

Muscles: Glutes, hamstrings, lower back.

Sets: 3 **Reps:** 8

- Stand with feet together and hands at the sides.

- Bend forward at the hips, raising one leg off the ground while tipping the upper body forward towards the ground.

- Reach forward with the same side arm as the raised leg and touch the ground.

- Pull the grounded heel to return to the start position.

- Complete all repetitions before switching sides.

- Keep the shoulders pulled back with butt, thighs, and abs tight to maintain body position throughout the exercise.

- Regression: instead of raising the back leg off the ground, slide it back along the floor until the body is at a 45-degree angle, pull back through the heel.

- Progression: perform the exercise on a cushion. This will challenge your balance.

Working the Core

Improving core strength can lead to a myriad of benefits for health, movement, and appearance. The core muscles are directly involved with lung function, and their development will lead directly to deeper and easier breathing. Any abdominal cramps experienced with intense exercise are core muscles seizing, as they are not used to the currently applied load. Deeper breathing allows for stress relief, better sleep, and possibly even fat loss due to more intense workouts and decreased cortisol, a stress hormone that promotes fat retention.

Exercises can be performed in supersets, groups of three exercises, or a full circuit.

Plank

Muscles: Abs, lower back, glutes.

Sets: 3 **Reps:** 30 seconds

- Lie face down on the floor with toes tucked under the feet held together; elbows and forearms are tucked at the side with hands pointed straight ahead.

- Push the body up so that elbows are directly under the shoulders, forearms, and toes are on the ground, and the body is straight.

- Pinch the thighs, butt, and abs and hold for a count of three.

- Don't allow the hips to drop or the back to the curve at any time.

- **Regression:** perform with feet held shoulder width apart or on the knees.

- **Progression:** a leg or arm can be taken off the ground, or the opposite arm and leg held off the ground (most difficult).

Prone Raise

Muscles: Abs, glutes, lower back.

Sets: 3 **Reps:** 5 per arm

- Begin in a push-up position.

- Keep the back flat and tighten the thighs, butt, and abs throughout the set.

- Take one hand off the ground and extend it in front of the head until parallel to the floor.

- Pause at the top of the movement before returning to the starting position.

- Repeat the movement with the other arm.

- **Regression:** the feet can be widened, the hands can be raised to the side instead of in front, or the exercise can be performed on the knees.

- **Progression:** the feet can be brought closer together, or the opposite leg can be raised while raising the arm.

Reverse Crunch

Muscles: Abs, obliques, lower back.

Sets: 3 **Reps:** 8

- Lie flat on the floor on your back.

- Fully extend your legs and place your hands flat on the floor beside you.

- Draw your knees up towards your chest while keeping your feet together.

- Hold for a count of three.

- In a controlled movement, return to the start position.

- Repeat

- **Regression:** place your arms behind your head.

- **Progression:** hold the arms up, fingers pointing straight up in the air.

Side Plank

Muscles: Abs, oblique, triceps, deltoids.

Sets: 3 **Reps:** 15 seconds per side

- Lie on your side with feet stacked on each other, elbow directly under the shoulder and forearm against the ground perpendicular to the rest of the body.

- Lift the hips off the ground until the body is in a straight line.

- The top shoulder should be directly above the lower shoulder, with both shoulders pulled back.

- The thighs, butt, and abs are tight throughout to ensure that the spine is held straight.

- **Regression:** perform with knees stacked on the ground.

- **Progression:** raise the top leg off the grounded leg.

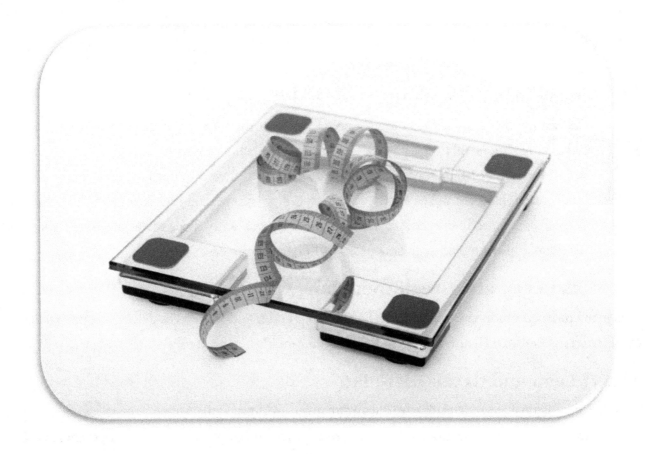

PROGRAMS OF THE LEAN AND GREEN DIET

The Lean and Green Diet encourages people to limit the number of calories that they should take daily. Under this program, dieters are encouraged to consume between 800 and 1,000 calories daily. For this to be possible, dieters are encouraged to opt for healthier food items and meal replacements. But unlike other types of commercial diet regimens, the Lean and Green diet comes in different variations. There are currently three variations of the Lean and Green diet plan that one can choose according to their needs.

5&1 Lean and Green Diet Plan

This is the most common version of the Lean and Green diet, and it involves eating five pre-packaged meals from the Optimal Health Fuelings and one home-made balanced meal.

4&2&1 Lean and Green Diet Plan

This diet plan is designed for people who want to have flexibility while following this regimen. Under this program, dieters are encouraged to eat more calories and have more flexible food choices. This means that they can consume 4 pre-packaged Optimal Health fuelings food, two home-cooked meals from the lean and green, and one snack daily.

5&2&2 Lean and Green Diet Plan

This diet plan is perfect for individuals who prefer to have a flexible meal plan to achieve a healthy weight. It is recommended for a wide variety of people. Under this diet regimen, dieters must eat 5 fuelings, 2 lean and green meals, and 2 healthy snacks.

3&3 Lean and Green Diet Plan

This particular diet plan is created for people who have moderate weight problems and merely want to maintain a healthy body. Under this diet plan, dieters are encouraged to consume 3 pre-packaged Optimal Health fuelings and three home-cooked meals.

Lean and Green for Nursing Mothers

This diet regimen is designed for nursing mothers with babies of at least two months old. Aside from supporting breastfeeding mothers, it also encourages gradual weight loss.

Lean and Green for Diabetes

This Lean and Green diet plan is designed for people who have type 1 and type 2 diabetes. The meal plans are designed to consume more green and lean meals, depending on their needs and condition.

Lean and Green for Gout

This diet regimen incorporates a balance of foods that are low in purines and moderate in protein.

Lean and Green for Seniors (65 years and older)

Designed for seniors, this Lean and Green diet plan has some variations following the components of fuelings depending on the senior dieters' needs and activities.

Lean and Green for Teen Boys and Lean and Green for Teen Girls (13–18 years old)

Designed for active teens, the Lean and Green for teen boys and Lean and Green for teen girls provide the right nutrition to growing teens.

Regardless of which type of Lean and Green diet plan you choose, you must talk with a coach to determine which plan is right for you based on your individual goals.

How to Start This Diet

The Lean and Green diet is comprised of different phases. A certified coach will educate you on the steps that you need to undertake if you want to follow this regimen. Below are some things you need to know, especially when you are still starting with this diet regimen.

Initial Steps

During this phase, people are encouraged to consume from 800 to 1,000 calories to help you shed off at least 12 pounds within the next 12 weeks. For instance, if you are following the 5&1 Lean and Green diet plan, you need to eat 1 meal every 2 or 3 hours and include a 30-minute moderate workout on most days of your week. You need to consume not more than 100 grams of carbs daily during this phase.

Further, consuming meals are highly encouraged. This phase also encourages the dieter to include 1 optional snack per day, such as ½ cup sugar-free gelatin, 3 celery sticks, and 12 ounces nuts. Aside from these things, below are other things that you need to remember when following this phase:

- Make sure that the portion size recommendations are for cooked weight and not the raw weight of your ingredients.

- Opt for meals that are baked, grilled, broiled, or poached. Avoid fried foods, as this will increase your calorie intake.

- Eat at least 2 servings of fish rich in omega-3 fatty acids. These include fishes like tuna, salmon, trout, mackerel, herring, and other cold-water fishes.

- Choose meatless alternatives like tofu and tempeh.

- Follow the program even when you are dining out. Keep in mind that drinking alcohol is discouraged when following this plan.

Maintenance Phase

As soon as you have attained your desired weight, the next phase is the transition stage. It is a 6-week stage that involves increasing your calorie intake to 1,550 per day. This is also when you can add more varieties into your meal, such as whole grains, low-fat dairy, and fruits.

After six weeks, you can now move into the 3&3Lean and Green diet plan, so you are required to eat 3 lean and green meals and 3 fueling foods.

How Easy Is to Follow Lean and Green Diet

Practicing the Lean and Green diet gives you an option of about 60 Fuelings, but that is not to say you will still not have yearnings for other food options, especially those you are used to before taking up the diet plan.

All the recipes are readily available, and you can also take the option of dining out by following your guide. However, alcohol consumption is prohibited. You can order your meals easily or prepare them in your kitchen in a few minutes. You can easily get the needed tools to make your meals from your coach or request help from the online community.

You can get various ideas for your lean and green meals by visiting the brand Pinterest page. You will also get a recipe conversion guide that you can use whenever you have trouble with your recipe measurement.

You might face many challenges whenever you decide to eat out. However, it is not impossible to eat out. The brand advised you to let your lean and green meals be the only option when considering eating out to be on the safe side. By going through the dining out guide, you will know how to navigate buffets, order beverages, and select condiments and toppings for your meals.

It is straightforward to choose a plan and make your order that will be delivered instantly. Food preparation is swift, and the only area where you can face difficulty is adding water and nuking in the microwave. Anyone with no knowledge of cooking can easily tackle and get over the preparation of preparing the meals without breaking a sweat.

The Lean and Green coaches aim to help you adopt healthy habits. You will get weekly and monthly support calls from the Lean and Green coaches. Once you are a community member, you will also be able to partake in community events and have access to the nutrition support team, mainly composed of dietitians. Informational guides and FAQs can also be accessed online easily and for free.

The company says the recommended meals have a high "fullness index," which means that the high protein and fiber contents should help you to get satisfied for an extended period.

The meals you will be taking are tailored for the weight and fat loss purpose and may not win a cuisine competition. It is pertinent to note that the Lean and Green fuelings you will feed on will not contain flavors, artificial colors, or sweeteners.

No matter the plan you pick out, you start by using having a smartphone communique with a coach to help you determine which Lean and Green plan to follow, set weight loss desires, and make yourself familiar with the application.

Eating out can be challenging but still possible. If you love eating out, you can download Lean and Green's dining out guide. The guide comes with tips on how to navigate buffets, order beverages, and choose condiments. Aside from following the guide, you can also ask the chef to make substitutions for the ingredients used in cooking your food. For instance, you can ask the chef to serve no more than 7 ounces of steak and serve it with steamed broccoli instead of baked potatoes.

Opt for lean and green foods that have high fullness index. Eat foods that contain high protein and fiber content as they can keep you full for longer periods. Many nutrition experts highlight the importance of satiety when it comes to weight loss.

You have access to knowledgeable coaches. If you follow the Lean and Green diet plan, you can access knowledgeable coaches and become a part of a community that will give you access to support calls and community events. You also have a standby nutrition support team that can answer your questions.

No matter what diet plan you pick, begin by having a teleconference with a certain coach to determine which Lean and Green diet plan to follow, establish weight loss objectives, and acquaint yourself with the platform.

What to Eat

Depending on the type of diet plan you choose, you have to eat a number of lean and green meals comprised mainly of lean proteins and non-starchy vegetables. Although this diet regimen is not as restrictive as other diet regimens, there are plenty of foods compliant with this diet, including healthy fats. Thus, below are the types of foods that you can eat while following the Lean and Green diet.

Lean meats: Lean and green meals require you to make foods out of lean meats. There are three categories of lean meats identified by Lean and Green, including (1) lean, (2) leaner, and (3) leanest. Lean meats include salmon, pork chops, and lamb, while leaner meats include chicken breasts and swordfish. Leanest meats include egg whites, shrimp, and cod.

Green and non-starchy vegetables: Non-starchy vegetables are further identified as (1) lower carb, (2) moderate carb, and (3) higher carb. Lower carbs include all types of salad greens and green leafy vegetables. Moderate carb vegetables include summer squash and cauliflower. Lastly, high carb vegetables include peppers and broccoli.

Healthy fats: Healthy fats are encouraged for people who follow the Lean and Green diet. These include healthy fats such as olive oil, walnut oil, flaxseed, and avocado. However, it is important to consume two healthy fats to still keep up with the Lean and Green diet.

Others: Once dieters can achieve their weight-loss goals through meal replacements, they can start consuming other foods to maintain their ideal weight. These include low-fat dairy, fresh fruits, and whole grains. You can also consume meatless alternatives, including 2 cups egg substitute and 5 ounces seitan. For low-fat dairy, you are allowed to consume 1 ½ cups 1% cottage cheese, and 12 ounces of non-fat Greek yogurt

What Not to Eat

Similar to other diet regimens, the Lean and Green Diet also discourages dieters not to eat certain types of foods. This section will discuss the foods that are non-compliant to the principles of the Lean and Green Diet.

Indulgent Desserts

This diet regimen discourages the consumption of indulgent desserts such as cakes, ice cream, cookies, and all kinds of pastries. While eating these foods is discouraged during the first few weeks of following the diet, moderate consumption of sweet treats such as fresh fruits and yoghurts can be integrated into one's diet.

Sugary Beverages

Similar to indulgent desserts, sugary beverages are also discouraged among those who follow the Lean and Green Diet. These include soda, fruit juices, and energy drinks.

Unhealthy Fats

Fats such as butter, shortening, and commercial salad dressings contain large amounts of calories that are not good for people who are trying to lose weight. Moreover, they also contain preservatives and salt that is not good for the overall health.

Alcohol

Those who follow the Lean and Green Diet should limit their alcohol intake to 5 ounces of alcohol daily.

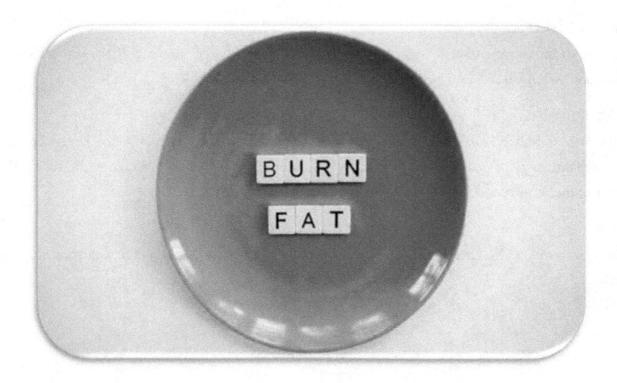

WHY WILL YOU LOSE WEIGHT IN CRITICAL AREAS?

The Lean and Green diet is a very effective tool for weight loss since you will be feeding on a meager 800-1,000 calories per day, which is about a 50% reduction of an adult recommended calorie daily intake.

The Company carried out a 16-week survey on their customers taking the Lean and Green diet program. They realized that participants of the 5&1 plan that were either obese or have excess weight had a significantly lower waist circumference, fat levels, and overall general weight than participants undergoing the weight maintenance plan (3&3 plan). The study also emphasizes the need for participants to take the coaching session very important. It shows that participants of the 5&1 plan that attended not less than 75% of their coaching session lost twice as much weight as those outside the range.

Lean and Green diet has the rank number #22 in the Easiest Diets to Follow. With the diet, you will get up to 60 Fueling options, but it might be quite difficult not to yearn for a different food option while on a diet. But one good thing is that you can eat as much as 6 times a day, which means only a few hour difference would be among your meals, and you do not need to count carbs, calories, or points—you are practically not going to be tracking anything!

With the varieties of recipes that you can choose from and eating out with the dining guide that would be provided for you after enrolling in the diet program, taking the Lean and Green diet is possible for almost anyone. Preparing meals or ordering meals online is also very fast; hence, you can still take the diet program conveniently if you are a busy type. Although it is recommended that your lean and green meals should be the meals you should eat. However, drinking alcohol is highly discouraged.

The meals you will be eating while on the Lean and Green diet have been shown to have a high "fullness index," which implies that you will get satiety after taking each meal. Even though the meals will have zero chance of winning in any cuisine competitions, the *Lean and Green "fuelings"* are devoid of sweeteners, flavors, or colors.

Exercise requirements

With the Lean and Green diet, you do not need to engage in high-intensity exercises. However, the company recommends moderate-intensity exercise like walking, which should be for 30 minutes daily. You are expected not to go overboard with the exercises to preserve your energy. If you are on the Optimal Weight 5&1 Plan, your coach will brief you on the recommended exercises you can engage in, but bear in mind that exercises are not an integral part of the Lean and Green diet program.

With the Lean and Green diet, you will have to eat portion-controlled meals and recommended snacks, which will ultimately help you lose weight. Your calories and carbs intake would be significantly reduced. With 800–1,000 calories divided between 6 portion-controlled meals daily on the 5&1 plan, and studies backing up, lowering calorie intake effectively decreases fat and weight loss.

One-on-one coaching is also instrumental in achieving weight loss, as studies have shown a significant improvement in losing weight to diet programs that usually include coaching sessions. It is pertinent to note that there is a high tendency to gain some weight after you are done with the 5&1 plan; for that reason, you should opt for the maintenance phase for the 3&3 plan.

Steps to Optimal Health

On the off chance that you flourish with structure and need to get more fit rapidly, the Lean and Green diet could be a solid match for you.

Before you start any feast substitution diet, cautiously consider whether you can sensibly tail it, choose how much cash you can contribute, and decide the level of craving and interference to your social routine you are alright with.

On the off chance that you choose to settle on Lean and Green and prevail with your transient weight-loss objectives, ensure you become taught about smart dieting so you can keep the weight off the long haul.

Let me share a little something I have learned in our Lean and Green Community before we end. It is called the six steps to optimal health. This is to ensure that you will fully and successfully embark on your journey in doing this diet.

The Lean and Green diet plan community suggests inspiration and real responses alongside the path to vitality, health, and confidence. It is all constructed on our community, 6-steps method that will empower you to reach your specific goals and build your footing for optimal lifetime health.

Prepare for Your Journey

As you take your first step toward a healthier life, your Lean and Green coach will be there for you to help you see what's possible and work with you to set the right goals for yourself. For most people, learning the lifestyles leading to optimal health commences with accomplishing a healthy weight.

Talk to your chosen or available coach or coaches about:

- Any questions you have about starting your journey.

- Learning the habits of Health Transformational System.

- Helping you complete your well-being evaluation online.

- Guiding you to set goals for your health and wellness.

Achieve a Healthy Weight

A healthy weight is a catalyst for bigger changes, and the Optimal Weight 5&1 plan is the way to get there:

- You need to remember to work side-by-side with your chosen Lean and Green coach to surely follow the proven 5&1 Optimal Weight plan included in this guide.

- Notice and rejoice each victory, however small it may seem, and talk over new opportunities with your chosen Lean and Green coach.

- Partake in the weekly community support teleconferences.

- Recognize and take charge of your energy organization system.

Transition to Healthy Eating

When you know what optimal nutrition appears like, healthy eating develops into your second nature. Work with your Lean and Green coach to compute a calorie consumption level that preserves your new healthy weight. Our 3&3 Optimal Health diet plan comprises of 3 Optimal Health fuelings and 3 well-balanced meals per day. Kindly continue to adore your favored Lean and Green fuelings or mix it up, whatever works best with your lifestyle. Select the right serving sizes and start upping your total energy spending, also referred to as the calories you burned daily, by moving more. Visit the Lean and Green website for the energy spending calculator and healthy guilt-free meal plans curated by our registered and expert dietitians. Increasing your activity is also an important part of maintaining a healthy weight. Also, do not forget that your Lean and Green coach is always around for any amount of support.

Live the Habits of Health

The more you include healthy practices into every little thing you do, the healthier you may appear and feel. The following modifications develop into a positive part of your routine. Next, you will know the habits of Healthy Motion and habits of Healthy Sleep, all in partnership with an Lean and Green coach.

Optimize Health for Your Age

You have taken the introductory Habits of Health. Tiny victories are accumulating up to big ones. You are feeling more confident, healthier, and your energy levels are up. You have positively incorporated the Habits of Health into your lifestyle.

Another aspect of your lifelong conversion is optimization. Handling stress and shaping your life around is what matters most to you. This is when you see that what commenced as a voyage to optimal health can become an influential opportunity. Your conversion can motivate other people as you level up from being coached to be a coach. You are building a successful and growing business while showing others the path to optimal health. Undoubtedly, you can become a leader in the community.

The Potential to Live a Longer, Healthier Life

No one can predict how long you are going to live. Still, research suggests that making an overall lifestyle change by taking an active role in your selections and performance, including eating healthier, reducing stress, losing weight, and moving more, can help you live a longer and healthier life.

An optimum life means remaining as fit as you can, for the longest time possible. After all, with transformed health and energy, your life can turn into whatever you desire it to be.

Optimal health is designated by healthy weight, healthy sleep, health habits, the desire to get better, and healthy motion.

You are reaching for ultra health.

You are learning how to develop ultimate energy control.

You are learning to help protect brain function and support a healthy body.

Following the Lean and Green Diet

The developers of the Lean and Green Diet strives to be transparent when developing their many regimens and plans. But if you have questions about this diet regimen, below are some FAQs that many people ask.

Which Lean and Green Diet Plan Is Good for Me?

As there are so many diet plans offered by Lean and Green, it is important to get in touch with a certified Lean and Green coach to learn about the many options you have. You must not make a second guess of the diet plan you will follow as each diet plan is designed to fit a particular profile. For instance, if you are a very active person, you can take on the Lean and Green 5&1 plan. But then, the coach will also look at other factors such as your age and health risks so that you can be matched with the right Lean and Green diet plan.

Can I Skip the Fuelings?

No. You must stick with fuelings if you want to follow the Lean and Green diet successfully. Fuelings are designed to provide the body with balanced amounts of macronutrients to promote an efficient fat-burning state to help people lose fat without losing energy. If you skip fueling, you may miss out on important nutrients that might lead to fatigue while following this diet. The body feels fatigued because it cannot compensate for the lack of nutrients while being calorie deficient.

Can I Rearrange My Fuelings?

Yes. If you are a busy person with a dynamic schedule, you can rearrange the timing when you will take your fueling meals. The Lean and Green diet is not strict about rearranging meals as long as you consume your meals within 24 hours. This versatility on your eating schedule makes it perfect for people who also have unusual schedules, including those who work at night or beyond regular working hours. So how do you time your fuelings? Just make sure that you eat your meals every two or three hours throughout the time that you are awake. Your first meal should be taken an hour after waking up to ensure optimal blood sugar levels. This is also great for hunger control.

Can I Rearrange My Fuelings, Especially If I Work on Long Days or Night Shifts?

Yes. You can rearrange the timing of your fuelings depending on your schedule. What is important is that you consume your fuelings and lean and green meals within 24 hours. So, whether you work at night or on regular hours, make sure that you eat your meals every 2 or 3 hours throughout the time that you are awake.

How Often Should I Eat My Meals?

The Lean and Green diet plan teaches you the habit of eating healthy. You are encouraged to eat six small meals daily. As mentioned earlier, you are encouraged to eat every two to three hours from your waking time. Thus, start your day with fuelings and eat your lean and green meals in between your fuelings. It is recommended that you eat your first meal within an hour of waking to ensure optimal blood sugar. This is also a good strategy for hunger control.

How to build your own Lean and Green Meal

A lean and green meal is made of 5 to 7 oz. of a lean protein of your choice. The more the protein is "lean" the more ounces you are allowed to eat.

In addition to that, you have to incorporate a quantity of healthy fats, depending by how much lean is your protein.

Lastly, you have to add the vegetables. Depending on how much carbohydrates are contained in a vegetable, this is classified in High, Medium or Low Carb. The lower the carbohydrate, the higher the quantity allowed to eat.

It may sound complicated but if you follow the tables below you will find that it is easier than expected. I hope you find them useful and that they will allow you to create a thousand healthy and delicious recipes!

Proteins for each lean and green meal

type	example	quantity	allowed servings of healthy fat
lean	salmon	5oz	0
	tuna		
	farmed catfish		
	herring		
	mackerel		
	lean beef		
	lamb		
	pork fillet		
	chicken tighs		
	turkey tighs		
	tofu	15oz	
	eggs	3	
	ricotta part-	8oz	

skim cheese		
tempeh	5oz	
part-skim cheese	4oz	
leaner	SWORDFISH	
		6oz
		1
halibut		
trout		
chicken breast (no skin - 94% lean)		
turkey breast (no skin - 94% lean)		
eggs	2	
egg whites	4	
2% cottage cheese	12oz or 1 cup	
low fat greek yogurt	12oz	
leanest	COD	
		7oz
		2

haddock	
flounder	
orange	
roughy	
tilapia	
grouper	
haddock	
mahi	
mahi	
wild	
catfish	
tuna	
(canned	
in water)	
scallops	
crab	
lobster	
shrimp	
game	
meat	
ground	
turkey	
breast	
(98%	
lean)	
egg	14 or
whites	2
	cups
seitan	5oz
1%	2oz
cottage	or 1
cheese	½
	cups
no fat	12oz

greek

yogurt

healthy fats – 1 serving

example	quantity
oil (extra-virgin olive oil would be recommended)	1 tbsp.
reduced-fat, low-carbohydrate salad dressing	2 tbsp.
black or green olives	5-10
avocado	1 ½
nuts (almonds, peanuts or pistachios)	⅓ oz.
seeds (sesame, chia, flax or pumpkin seeds)	1 tbsp.
butter, margarine, mayonnaise	½ tbsp.

Greens for each lean and green meal

type	example	quantity
high carb	red cabbage	
		1 ½ cup
	squash	
	collard	
	chayote squash (cooked)	
	green or wax beans	
	broccoli	
	kabocha squash	
	leeks (cooked)	
	kohlrabi	
	okra	
	peppers	
	scallions	
	summer squash	
	turnips	
	tomatoes	
	cores	
	jicama	
	swiss chard	
moderate carb	CABBAGE	
	eggplant	
	cauliflower	1 ½
	fennel bulb	cup
	asparagus	
	mushrooms	
	kale	
	portabella	
	zucchini	
	spinach (cooked)	
low carb	ENDIVE	

green leaf lettuce	
butterhead	3
romaine	cup
iceberg	
collard (fresh/raw)	
spinach (fresh/raw)	
mustard greens	
watercress	
bok choy (raw)	
spring mix	
cucumbers	
radishes	
white mushrooms	1 ½
sprouts	cup
turnip greens	
celery	
arugula	
escarole	
swiss chard (raw)	
jalapeno (raw)	
bok choy (cooked)	
nopales	

Condiment

Condiments can add more flavor to each meal or fueling you consume and, ultimately, can make the whole process more enjoyable. It is fundamental that you develop a healthy awareness of them so they can become your allies to achieve a long-term transformation. That's why I recommend to always remember that they add up to your carbohydrates intake and to always read the labels so you can correctly dose them. The golden rule is that you can consume three servings of condiment per day in the 5&1 plan. Each serving must provide no more than 1 gram of carbohydrate per serving.

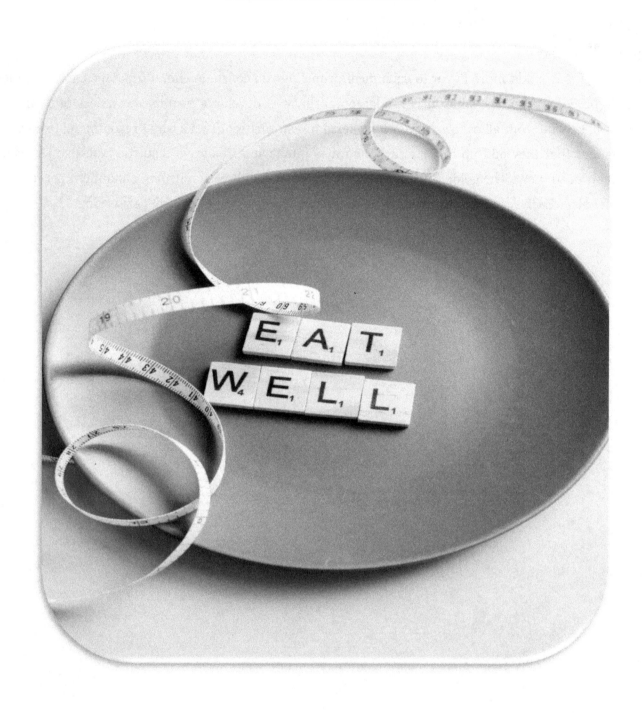

WHAT TO DO IN FRONT OF AN INVITATION TO DINNER?

What You Benefit from These Lean and Green Diet Recipes?

I f you find yourself going off and on a rollercoaster eating habit, you definitely should try out the recipes outlined in this book. Lean and Green diet comes with a structure and organization that's needed to get you off on a good start and take you to your desired destination if you follow it well. Anyway, the account of my friends simply portrays that some discipline is, of course, required. Even if you're an emotional eater or a binge eater, the Lean and Green diet encourages you to exercise a bit of control.

The diet is a high-protein diet and typically makes up about 10–35% of your daily calorie intake. The protein serves as a carb alternative when your body needs energy. On average, your calorie intake per day may hover around 800–1,000 as the Lean and Green diet relies on the intense restriction of calories and active promotion of weight loss. The calories of most fuelings are around 100–110 each.

Lean and Green diets encourage you to do away with junk by eating nutrition-rich fuelings and making your food based on a healthy template. If you are often too busy to cook, the diet allows for a varying degree of flexibility when it comes to preparing your meal, as well as a complementary degree of pre-packaged foods or fuelings to go with your cooking timetable. In essence, following the program is a no brainer as a structure has been provided for you. For individuals seeking to achieve weight loss through healthy eating, the recipes included serves just that purpose, but your eating plan will depend on whether you're watching your weight or trying to reduce your weight. Whatever the case, the plans are simple and detailed. The coaching and community support help you to adhere to the structure of the program.

In case you didn't know, the fuelings are the features that make Lean and Green recipes stand out among many other weight loss programs. The fuelings are made without artificial additives, colors, or sweeteners. In addition to that, their "select" line is preservative-free. Although the meals are mostly pre-packaged, especially for the first two levels, they still do not contain any stimulants and no wacky pills or supplements. Emphasis is instead placed on regular eating of small portions of meals and snacks each day.

Also, the recipes are simple and easy to make, so you don't have to worry about spending too much time in the kitchen.

Following The Lean and Green Diet

To begin with, you'll need to make up your mind on which Lean and Green diet plan to go for. However, you can consult with the program coach if you're having trouble deciding which plan is best for you. You may also get assistance from your nutritionist. This is important to ensure that you get the best out of the program. For instance, most people who intend to pursue an intensive weight loss diet usually begin with the Lean and Green 5&1 plan, which caps your daily intake of calories is at 1,000. Reports from several pieces of research show that enrollees can shed up to about 12 pounds within 12 weeks of starting the program. The plan allows you to eat 5 fuelings or pre-packaged meals and snacks and one low-calorie home-made (lean and green meal) each day at a spacing of 2–3 hours. In addition to that, followers are encouraged to incorporate a 30-minutes exercise routine up to 4 times a week.

The lean and green meals can be made at home but can also be ordered from the Lean and Green brand at an additional cost. But if you're not too busy to make meals at home, and if you wish to avoid the extra cost of purchasing the lean and green meals, you can rely on the easy-to-apply process and recipes that we've included in this book to get you going smoothly. Remember, the 5&1 plan includes one optional snack per day. You can rely on any of the suggestions provided in our recipes or simply order one from your coach. If you must eat out, you're better off with the guidance of a coach or nutrition expert. Better still, you can enquire to be sure that the food does not contradict the Lean and Green diet in content.

The Maintenance Phase

The optimal weight 4&2&1 plan is designed for this stage of weight loss. You may begin using the recipes outlined for this plan once you reach your desired weight. Practically, you'll enter a transition phase that allows you to slowly increase your calorie intake up to 1,500 calories per day. It is more flexible and less restrictive than the first phase. As you'll find in the listed recipes, you can add a variety of other foods, such as whole grains and fruits, to your daily intake.

The final phase of the Lean and Green diet allows for even more flexibility in terms of what you can eat. The 4&2&1 plan is designed to last for up to 6 weeks, after which you may proceed to the final phase - the optimal health 3&3 plan. Here, the fuelings and lean and green meals are apportioned equally. 3 fuelings and 3 lean and green meals daily. At this stage, you must have achieved the desired weight and are ready to transition off the program. At the same time, you would have been properly re-orientated towards a healthier eating habit. As you move on to traditional meals, you're armed with a better idea of what an ideal food is. Also, note that alcohols do not work with the Lean and Green diet, and you have to take exercises seriously to ensure that you have sustainable change

Tips for Dining Out

One of the main downsides of following a dietary regimen is that you have to give up a little your social life.

It is difficult to enjoy a happy hour or a dinner out with your girlfriends if you follow a strict protocol and this limitation can sometime be the reason why many people give up diet in the first place.

Luckily, by following the instruction on the paragraph above you can still enjoy a dinner out with your friends at your favorite restaurant. You have only to choose the right foods from the menu or gently ask to the waiter for a custom dish.

In addition, we would like to recommend the following when dining out:

- No alcohol: Alcoholic beverages are mainly empty calories. Moreover they promote dehydration and fog your mind, causing a potential fall into not allowed foods

- Carefully research the menu before you go to the restaurant (by searching on the internet), find the right food for you and stick to them (no dessert alloed!)

- Choose the right people: be sure to go out with people who support you and your transformational journey

- Eat mindfully: not only you will enjoy your food more but you will also increase your satiation level

- Be engaged in the conversation: you went out to stay with your friends and enjoy their company in the first place. Never forget it!

- Don't go hungry: drink plenty of water before going and try to move the fuelings closer to the dinner time so you will not be so hungry

- Practice portion control: stick to the right quantity of foods for your needs.

Tips to deal with Cravings

Changing habits is never an easy task, and you may find yourself wandering near the fridge during the first days of your Lean and Green journey.

The good news is: you are not alone: here some tips to stay on track:

- Brush your teeth and use mouthwash

- Distract yourself with intense mental activity such as a puzzle

- Exercise or go for a walk outside

- Avoid the situations that trigger your cravings

- Drink more water Pros and Cons of Lean and Green Diet

The Lean and Green diet depends on restrictive dinner substitution items and carefully calorie-controlled arranged suppers, so there's very little space for change.

The 5&1 plan limits calories to as low as 800–1,000 every day, so it is not appropriate for women who are pregnant or individuals participating in exercises that require maximum physical activity.

Extraordinary calorie limitation can cause exhaustion, mind haze, cerebral pains, or menstrual changes. Al things considered, the 5&1 alternative ought not to be utilized long haul.

Be that as it may, the 3&3 and 4&2&1 plan normally gracefully between 1,100 to 2,500 calories for every day and can be fitting to use for a more extended period.

Pros

Lean and Green 's program may be a solid match for you on the off chance that you need a diet plan that is clear and simple to follow, which will assist you with getting in shape rapidly, and offers worked in social help.

When embarking on any new diet regimen, you may experience some difficulties along the way. Below are the reasons why this diet regimen is considered the easiest to follow among all commercial diet regimens.

Accomplishes Rapid Weight Loss

Most solid individuals require around 1,600 to 3,000 calories per day to keep up their weight. Limiting that number to as low as 800 basically ensures weight loss for a great many people.

Lean and Green 's 5&1 plan is intended for brisk weight loss, making it a strong choice for somebody with a clinical motivation to shed pounds quickly.

You enter the fat-loss stage in just 3 days. Look for a weight loss story on YouTube to see how many people out there are losing an impressing amount of weight, even 20 or more pounds in a week.

The average of 12 pounds in 12 weeks on the website counts all the people that do it by themselves, and nobody knows how many times they actually follow the plan, how many times they cheat, how much water they drink, exercise, etc.

Easy to Follow

As the diet depends on generally pre-packaged fuelings, you are only accountable for doing one meal a day on the 5&1 Plan.

Moreover, each individual plan comes with meal logs and a sample meal plan to make it easier for the client to follow.

Although you are encouraged to make 1 to 3 lean and green foods a day, contingent on the strategy, they are very simple to make—because the program will include detailed recipes and a list of food options for you to choose from.

Also, those who are not keen on cooking can purchase pre-packaged meals called Flavors of Home to substitute for the lean and green meals.

Bundled Items Offer Comfort

Lean and Green 's shakes, soups, and all other feast substitution items are conveyed legitimately to your entryway—a degree of comfort that numerous different diets don't offer.

Although you should search for your own elements for lean and green dinners, the home conveyance choice for Lean and Green 's fuelings spares time and vitality.

When the items show up, they're anything but difficult to get ready and make phenomenal snatch and go suppers.

Packaged Products

They will be delivered directly at home, and they are quick-to-make and grab-and-go.

Eliminates the Guesswork

You don't need to worry about what to eat all day, cook just once a day or every other day.

A few people find that the hardest piece of dieting is the psychological exertion required to make sense of what to eat every day—or even at every supper.

It's Not a Ketogenic Diet

Carbs are allowed and higher than the majority of weight-loss diets out there, just not the refined ones.

No Counting Calories

You don't really need to count your calories when following this type of diet, just as long as you stick with the rule of fuelings, meals, snacks, and water intake depending on your preference may it be 5&1, 4&2&1, or 3&3.

Cons

There are additionally some potential drawbacks to Lean and Green 's plan, particularly on the off chance that you are stressed over cost, adaptability, and the assortment.

It's Tough the First Weeks

You may feel hungry in the first weeks; however, it will fade away soon.

Low Calories

Even though Lean and Green 's diet plan emphasizes frequently eating throughout the day, each of its fuelings only provides 110 calories. Lean and Green meals are also low in calories.

When you are eating fewer calories in general, you may find the plan leaves you hungry and unsatisfied. You may also feel more easily fatigued and irritable.

High Month-to-Month Cost

Lean and Green 's expense can be an obstacle for imminent clients.

The 5&1 plan goes in cost from $350 to $425 for 119 servings (around three weeks of dinner substitutions).

As you're thinking about the program's expense, remember to factor in the food you'll have to buy to set up your lean and green suppers.

Following picking your arrangement, you'll buy the food. Costs fluctuate and rely upon the amount you're purchasing (and what). It's frequently most straightforward to get one of their units. The Optimal Essential Kit, which sets with the 5&1 Optimal weight plan, accompanies 119 portions of food (counting shakes, sides, soups, bars, snacks, sides, and pasta) for only $414.60. The Optimal Health Kit for the 3&3 plan offers 130 food servings of comparative things for $333.

May be Incompatible with Other Eating Plans

The Lean and Green diet incorporates specific projects for veggie lovers, individuals with diabetes, and breastfeeding ladies. Moreover, around 66% of its items are affirmed sans gluten. In any case, alternatives are constrained for those on explicit diets.

For instance, Lean and Green fuelings are not appropriate for veggie lovers or individuals with dairy hypersensitivities because most choices contain milk.

Moreover, the fuelings utilize various fixings, so those with food hypersensitivities should peruse the names cautiously.

At long last, the Lean and Green program isn't suggested for pregnant ladies since it can't meet their dietary needs.

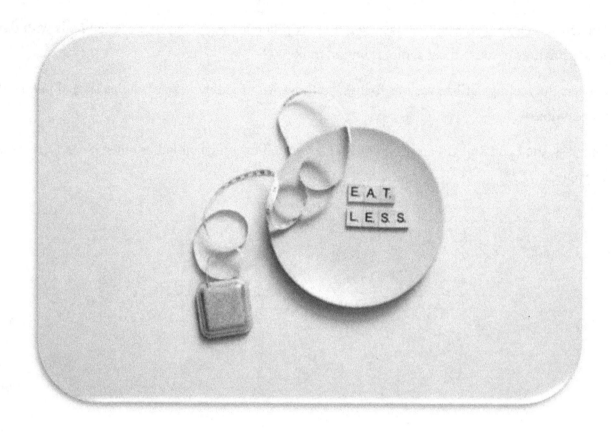

LEAN AND GREEN DIET IN THE KITCHEN

What Is Meal Prepping?

Meal prepping does not have to be something that you dread for each week. You can make it fun and involve the whole family. It always helps to have an extra hand along to keep up with everything. If you start eating the proper meals at the appropriate times, you are going to see the other benefits of eating healthy when you start losing weight and just feeling better mentally about yourself.

Meal prepping is exactly what the word says; it simply means that you prepare several meals or even all of them beforehand. Instead of eating ready-made meals which you would normally buy at a store you can now prepare your own. They will be better suited to your taste, contain fewer preservatives, and will be healthier.

The core part of success for meal prepping is that you must have a PLAN. You will not succeed if you do not have a plan. I can most certainly promise you that.

How to Meal Prep in a Few Easy Steps?

Once you are on the road to becoming good at meal prepping, you will never look back. You will very likely continue moving forward onto the next great set of healthy meal prep recipes!

Buy in Bulk

Where or whenever you can, always buy food supplies for meal preps in bulk. It is going to be a lot cheaper to do so, and it will certainly make it easier for you to decide on meals for the evening. You can meal prep some of it, then freeze the rest to use for another meal prep session, perhaps the following week.

Prioritize Your Meals

Do this especially when you do not have time to prepare all of them at once. You need to pick the most important meals to complete first. If you are someone that likes to have snacks, make sure that you chop plenty of fruits and veggies to snack on. This is preferable to doing a big meal prep when you are short of time.

Set Aside Time to Do Meal Prep

If you are cooking large batches, then you will need to put aside a day each week to get this done. Make sure that you are doing it when you do not feel rushed so that you can prepare the best meals possible.

Cook Large Batches of Food That You Are Fond of

You do not want to make a large batch of food only to find that it is not something that suits your taste. Try new recipes in small amounts before you decide to cook them in batches. Cook foods that you are familiar with at first in batches, then eventually expand to other new foods.

Slowly Build Up Food Variety

You do not have to cook 20 different food options in your first week. You can always start with one meal for dinner one day and have the leftovers for lunch the next day. It will take time to build up different options, so approach it slowly; don't feel rushed.

Bake Veggies & Meat on the Same Tray

You can save yourself fewer things to wash up by cooking your veggies and meat on one big tray in the oven. The juices will create a nice sauce that you can use on the meat to prevent it from going dry when you reheat it.

Make Some Smoothie-Cubes

Add smoothie mixture to the ice-cube tray, allow them to freeze, then add them all to a freezer bag. You can fill the ice-cube tray back up, repeat until you have filled your freezer bag with smoothie-cubes. Now you can take a couple of cubes out the night before and put them into a glass and some milk to water them down.

Multi-task

While you are cooking dinner, use the time that you are waiting for the food to finish cooking to chop up some veggies for your meals for the next few days. Once you get multi-tasking under your belt, you will find it much easier to get more things done within a shorter timeframe.

Spice Up Your Meals

Keep your meals full of flavor and interesting by adding spices to them. You can make your meal taste so much better just by adding some spices or allowing your meat to soak in a marinade.

Keep Prepping When You Can

Just keep in mind that anything that you do in the preparation of a meal ahead of time is considered meal prep. This includes chopping up veggies to cover you for the next few days.

Benefits of Planning Meals

Weight Loss

Meal prepping is going to **help you lose weight.** Knowing what you are going to eat is very important if you want to lose weight.

Finish Cravings

Cravings are going to stop as you continue to meal prep. In just a few weeks, you will find that you no longer crave sugar or junk. Instead, you will be looking forward to the meals and snacks that you have prepared.

Stress Is a Killer

It can cause so many problems with your health, such as increasing your blood pressure. It can cause sleep issues, lower your immune system, and even cause digestive problems.

No More Indecision

When you arrive home from work, exhausted and ravenous with hunger, and you will have a solution waiting for you. You open the cupboards, rummaging around while you wait for inspiration, but nothing springs to mind. With planning, this doesn´t happen.

No Worse Choices

Without a proper plan for your next meal, you may fall into the trap of going for the perceived 'easy option' of a takeaway or ready meal.

A More Balanced Diet

Take the time to think back on what exactly you have eaten the past week. You will probably realize that it was basically the same dish most of the time.

Much More Variety

Some people are of the opinion that planning your meals ahead of time is boring since you know what you are going to eat a few days in advance. This is far from the truth; planning actually encourages variety.

No Food Wastage While Saving Money

How often did you find wilted veggies in your refrigerator or had to throw away food that is past its expiry date? If you plan cleverly, making use of leftovers, using what is in your kitchen cupboards, freezing food in batches, very few food items will end up in your trashcan.

Less Arduous Arguing

You feel like a vegetarian dish; your partner wants hamburgers, but the kids plead for pizzas. Does this sound familiar? Your family may end up arguing unnecessarily over their next meal.

Go for Seasonal

Be clever and plan your meals according to the season. Not only will you have the freshest ingredients, but you will also look after your purse, as fresh items are cheaper when in season.

Saving Money

It is a huge misconception that healthy eating equals heavy spending. This is simply not true. There are many reasons why advance prepping can help you save money.

Must-Have Kitchen Essentials

Below are some of the essential kitchen equipment items that you might want to keep handy.

Cutting Boards

Try to get boards that are made from solid materials like plastic, glass, rubber, or marble. These are mostly corrosion-resistant, and the non-porous surface makes it easier to clean them than wood.

Measuring Cups

Required to measure out liquids, spices, and condiments.

Spoons

Have a number of different-sized spoons allow you to measure out small amounts of spices and other ingredients.

Glass Bowls and Non-Metallic Containers

These are required for storing items as well as for mixing ingredients.

Paper Towels

These are required for draining the food of excess oil and other liquids.

Cold Storage

Many fresh and cooked foods need to be stored at 40°F or below, so a refrigerator is required.

Knives

Knives should be used to slice meat, vegetables, fruit, and other food. While using the knife, you should keep the following in mind:

- Always use a sharp knife.

- Always keep your knives visible.

- Always cut down toward the cutting surface and away from your body.

- Never allow children to have unattended access to knives.

- Wash the knives often when cutting different types of food.

Kitchen Scales

A kitchen scale allows you to get accurate measurements of your ingredients, ideal for those following a diet plan.

Internal Thermometer

A meat thermometer helps you to measure the internal temperature of foods to ensure that they are safe to eat.

Baking Sheet

These are flat, rectangular metal pans that are used in an oven, ideal for roasting, baking, and keeping items warm.

Colander

A colander is a bowl-shaped kitchen utensil with holes that allows you to drain food like pasta. These are also used to rinse vegetables.

Aluminum Foil

This is used to wrap up and cover food and line baking sheets.

Parchment Paper

This is used to line baking sheets to help prevent items from sticking.

Storage Containers

These are the beating heart of meal prepping, so try to keep as many containers as possible. However, when selecting containers, you may notice there are two types of containers: plastic and glass.

Both have their merits and drawbacks. The following points should help you choose between the two.

Glass

- Glass containers are a bit more expensive but are ideal for long-term storage.

- Due to their heavyweight, glass containers are not ideal for "on-the-go" eating

- They are easier to clean.

- If you are concerned about plastic safety, then these are the ones to go with.

Plastic

- Easy to carry and lightweight, ideal for individuals who are always on the go.

- They are more convenient and come in a wide variety of sizes and shapes.

Asides from glass and plastic, you may also notice that there are steel containers. Steel containers are excellent if you want to keep meals in the freezer as they help to avoid freezer burn.

Amazing Meal Prep Ideas

Keep in mind that meal prep ideas are not set in stone. The following are just some of the dozens of different meal prep ideas that you are can find on the Internet.

- **Make a plan ahead of time:** If you are reading this book, then you have probably decided to go on a clean eating diet journey.

- **Keep a good supply of Mason jars:** Mason jars are terrific, not only for storing memories and canning foods but also for storing healthy salads.

- **Multiple seasonings in one pan:** If your diet requires you to stick with lean meats like chicken, then seasoning them as needed can become somewhat of a chore.

- **Boil eggs in an oven instead of a pot:** Now, this might sound a little bit odd at first, but it is highly effective.

- **Keep your prepared smoothies frozen in muffin tins:** The muffin tins can be useful here as well.

- **Roast vegetables that require the same time in one batch:** When you are preparing large batches of vegetables for roasting, go ahead and roast some extras at the same time.

- **Learn to use a skewer effectively:** When you think of skewers, you automatically think of kabobs.

- **Keep a good supply of sectioned plastic containers:** Sectioned containers are an absolute necessity for serious meal-prepping savants.

- **Keep track of your accomplishments:** This is perhaps the essential aspect of a meal-prepping routine.

The Common Mistakes Made by Meal Prepping Beginners

As a beginner in meal planning, you want to make sure that you are using your time wisely. You don't want to waste ingredients, waste time, or do other things that take away from the benefits that come with this kind of prep. Some of the common mistakes that you need to avoid as a beginner include:

Not Building a Balanced Meal

Eating too much of one food and not enough of another can mess up the day. The recipes below will help you to get the right balance between the carbs, protein, and fats that you need on the Lean and Green diet. But if you are choosing from other sources, make sure that you are balancing out the meals so that your macronutrients are still in place.

Preparing It All in One Day

It may be tempting to prepare all the food in one day, but have you ever tasted chicken, or other meat, after it has been in the fridge for a week? These often taste poorly, and you will not want to eat them. You can choose a few options. Some people just make meals for a few days at a time and call that good. If you need to make a lot of meals at once, consider freezing them to keep everything fresh for when you need it.

Never mixing it Up

Eating the same things or similar things can get boring. It is important to think about the meals that you are preparing and that you pick out a variety of meals that will taste good. Eating chicken every day for a month is boring, but mixing up the meals to include some fish, some beef, some turkey, and even some vegetarian options can make things easier.

Not Stocking Up the Kitchen

It is impossible to cook up these healthy meals without planning ahead a bit. If you are working on a recipe and you don't have the ingredients, you may reach for a substitute that is not that healthy. For example, you may need brown rice in a recipe and instead use white pasta when you are out. Always plan ahead and know what you need for all of your recipes to make things easier.

Not Storing Properly

The containers that you store the meals in can actually affect how much food you are going to make and eat. If you are picking out containers that are huge, your portion sizes are going to be large as well. Pick out portion-controlled containers, or ones that are only as big as the amount of food that your family will eat. You may find that some of the meals can be divided in two, saving you even more money.

Picking Out Complicated Cooking Methods

You do not need to pick out meals that are going to take hours to put together and need the most complicated cooking method possible. It is fine to keep things simple, especially when it comes to your meal planning. For example, there is nothing wrong with doing recipes each time that uses the slow cooker. You simply need to throw the ingredients in the slow cooker, and the meal is done. You can always mix it up with different cooking methods but making it simple is the name of the game with meal planning.

Tips and Tricks for Making Meal Prep Easy

What is great about these tips is that they are going to work for you, whether you are prepping your food just for you or for your entire family. What many people love about meal prep is that there is a huge community of people online that are sharing all of the recipes that they use, so there is no shortage of options.

- **Keep staples on hand.** Even if you are not prepping all of your meals, it is best to keep staples such as tempeh, boiled eggs, oatmeal, bananas, baked sweet potatoes, and shredded chicken on hand.

- **Make sure that your containers are functional.** Your containers are going to determine how successful you are at meal prepping.

- **Don't feel like you have to go on Pinterest and create the most complicated meals** because this is only going to lead to a bunch of Pinterest fails.

- **Practice makes perfect** when it comes to many things in life, including meal prepping.

- **Get to know your vegetables.** Not all vegetables are going to keep in the fridge for one week after they have been chopped.

- **Make sure that you plan your snacks and never leave the house without your water, snack, and meal** if you are going to be gone for long.

- **Make prepping a party.** Meal prep does take time; however, it is not a waste of time and should never be seen that way.

- **Cook all of the same foods at once.** One of the great things about meal prepping is that you can cook once and create several meals.

- **Purchase containers that are of proper proportion.**

- After prepping all of your meals, no one wants to spend even more time cleaning up.

- You can also clean as you go. If you spill something on the stove, wipe it up instead of letting it dry on and struggling to get it off later.

- **Purchase bags of frozen produce when possible.**

- **Make more than you will eat and then freeze the extra.**

- When you are first starting, **choose your trigger meal to prep.**

- If you are prepping all of your meals, don't forget to give yourself some variety.

- **Cook multiple foods at the same time.**

- **Once you have cooked all of your rice or quinoa, make sure that you use all of it.**

- There are so many ways for you to ensure your success as you are meal prepping, but the best tip that I can give you is to just keep at it.

- Meal prepping is not supposed to feel like a burden or another task that you have to complete, but instead, it is supposed to help you simplify your life while saving time and energy.

Advantages of Lean and Green Diet

The Lean and Green diet has extra advantages that may support weight reduction and general well-being.

Simple to Follow

As the diet depends for the most part on pre-packaged fuelings, you're just liable for preparing one dinner for every day on the 5&1 Plan.

Also, each arrangement accompanies supper logs and test dinner intends to make it simpler to follow.

While you're urged to cook 1–3 lean and green dinners every day, contingent upon the arrangement, they're easy to make—as the program incorporates explicit plans and a rundown of food alternatives.

May Improve Blood Circulatory

Lean and Green projects may help improve circulatory strain through weight reduction and restricted sodium consumption.

While the Lean and Green diet hasn't been explored explicitly, a 40-week concentrate in 90 individuals with overabundance weight or heftiness on a comparable Company program uncovered a huge decrease in circulatory strain.

Also, all Lean and Green feast plans are intended to give under 2,300 mg of sodium for every day—even though it's dependent upon you to pick low sodium choices for Lean and Green suppers.

Various well-being associations, including the Institute of Medicine, American Heart Association, and the United States Department of Agriculture (USDA), suggest expending under 2,300 mg of sodium each day.

That is because higher sodium admission is connected to an expanded danger of hypertension and coronary illness in salt-touchy people.

Offers Progressing Support

Lean and Green 's well-being coaches are accessible all through the weight reduction and upkeep programs.

As noted over, one investigation found a noteworthy connection between the quantity of instructing meetings on the Lean and Green 5&1 Plan and improved weight reduction.

Moreover, research proposes that having a way of life coach or advocate may help long haul weight support.

Potential Drawbacks of Lean and Green Diet

While the Lean and Green diet might be a successful weight reduction technique for a few, it has a few expected drawbacks.

Low in Calories

With only 800–1,2000 calories for every day, the Lean and Green 5&1 program is very low in calories, particularly for people who are accustomed to eating at least 2,000 every day.

While this fast decrease in calories may bring out general weight reduction, research has indicated that it can prompt huge muscle misfortune.

Moreover, low-calorie diets may diminish the number of calories your body consumes by as much as 23%. This more slow digestion can last significantly after you quit confining calories.

May be Hard to Stay with

The 5&1 Plan incorporates 5 pre-packaged fuelings and 1 low carb feast for each day. Accordingly, it very well may be very prohibitive in food choices and carbohydrate content.

As you may feel burnt out on depending on pre-packaged nourishments for the majority of your suppers, it could turn out to be anything but difficult to undermine the diet or create longings for different nourishments.

While the support plan is significantly less prohibitive, despite everything depends intensely on fuelings.

May Prompt Weight Regain

Weight recovery might be a worry after you stop the program.

Presently, no examination has inspected weight recapture after the Lean and Green diet. All things considered, in an investigation on a comparable, 16-week diet, members recovered a normal of 11 pounds (4.8 kg) inside 24 weeks of completing the program.

One likely reason for weight recovery is your dependence on bundled food things. After the diet, it might be hard to change to looking for and preparing solid suppers.

Moreover, because of the sensational calorie limitation of the 5&1 Plan, some weight recovery may likewise be because of more slow digestion.

Lean and Green Fuelings Are Profoundly Handled

The Lean and Green diet depends intensely on pre-packaged food things. Indeed, you would eat 150 pre-packaged fuelings every month on the 5&1 Plan.

This is a reason for worry; the same number of these things are profoundly prepared.

They contain a lot of food added substances, sugar substitutes, and prepared vegetable oils, which may hurt your gut well-being and add to constant aggravation.

Carrageenan, a typical thickener, and additive utilized in numerous fuelings, are gotten from red ocean growth. While research on its security is restricted, creature and test-tube contemplate proposing that it might contrarily influence stomach related well-being and cause intestinal ulcers.

Numerous fuelings likewise contain maltodextrin, a thickening specialist that has been appeared to spike glucose levels and harm your gut microbes.

While these added substances are likely sheltered in limited quantities, expending them much of the time on the Lean and Green diet may build your danger of symptoms.

The Program's Coach Is Not Well-Being Experts

Most Lean and Green coaches have effectively shed pounds on the program, however, are not confirmed, well-being experts.

Therefore, they are inadequate to give dietary or clinical exhortation. Hence, you should think about their direction while considering other factors and converse with your human services supplier if you have any worries. On the off chance that you have a current well-being condition, it's imperative to get the counsel of a clinical supplier or enlisted dietitian before beginning another diet program.

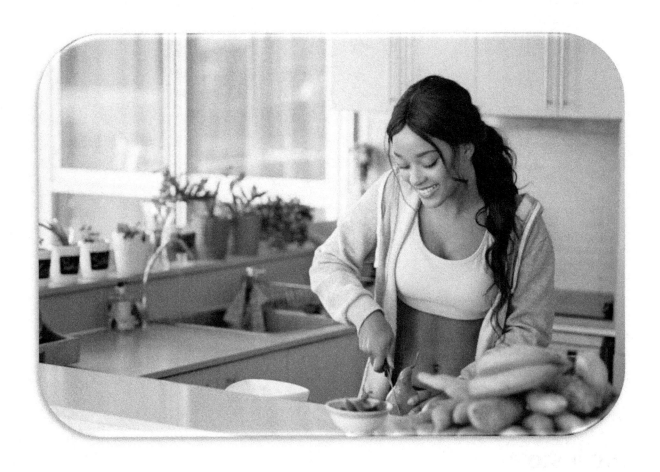

CONCLUSION

The logic behind the Lean and Green diet is that eating healthy recipes will make you feel full for a long time (not similarly to foods that are high in carbohydrates and saturated fat). That's why it focuses on increasing the consumption of whole foods and reducing dependence on fast commercial foods and other unhealthy foods.

The program has earned worldwide acclaim for its ability to deliver sustainable results without complicating the meal program for people. It places very few restrictions on food and inspires people to choose a healthier version of their daily food without compromising taste or nutrition.

Choosing the right diet or program had also become difficult as the industry flourished. Many diets claim to have specific health problems while helping a diet lose weight.

Unlike other diets, the Lean and Green diet is not designed for a specific health condition. It is designed according to the dieters' needs to achieve the ideal weight and the healthy lifestyle you want.

When you desire a structure and need to lose weight rapidly, the Lean and Green diet is the perfect solution.

The extremely low-calorie eating plans of the Lean and Green diet will definitely help you shed more pounds.

Before you start any meal replacement diet plan, carefully consider if it is truly possible for you to continue with a specific diet plan. When you have decided to stick with Lean and Green and make progress with your weight loss goal, ensure you have a brilliant knowledge about optimal health management to enable, and archive desired results effortlessly in the shortest time period.

The Lean and Green diet program is a stress-free and easy-to-follow program. It is a cool way to start a journey to your health.

Thank you!

LEAN AND GREEN COOKBOOK

2021

200 Recipes to Prepare Tasty, Easy, And Cheap Healthy Dishes for The Whole Family. Including Smoothies and Snacks for Definitive Weight Loss With 6 Meals Per Day

INTRODUCTION

The Lean and Green diet is based on the principles of eating many small meals a day, referred to as "Fuels," to always feel full and lose weight.

The rules of the Lean and Green diet are: eat every 2–3 hours; drink 1.5–2 liters of water per day; sleep at least 8 hours a night to reduce dietary stress; practice full-body training sessions (a type of training that exercises all muscle groups of the body) at least 20 minutes to half an hour a day, even at home; eat a total of 200 grams of protein foods per day, such as meat, fish, eggs, Greek yogurt, and skim cheeses; and consume 5 portions of fruit and vegetables a day.

The Lean and Green diet is possessed by a Company, a feast substitution organization. Its main diet and the Lean and Green one are low-calorie and low-carb programs that consolidate bundled foods with natively constructed dinners to energize weight reduction.

Effective weight-loss can often be a nightmare if you are following the wrong program. But you can also be certain that it works if you do the right thing. Lean and Green diet has been around for a while (though under a different name) and has been the saving hand for several people, including a couple of my friends.

If you are on the Lean and Green diet plan and need meal ideas for your daily consumption, this book will be a great buy.

If you are not on the Lean and Green diet, but you need low-carb meals to achieve quick weight loss, you can't be wrong with buying this book.

All the recipes in this book are centered on how you can lose weight quickly without counting calories, carbs, or points as all are naturally low in all of these and are geared towards achieving weight-loss.

HOW THE LEAN AND GREEN DIET WORKS?

Forms of the Eating Regimen

The Lean and Green diet incorporates two health improvement plans and a weight support plan, which are:

- **Ideal Weight 5&1 Plan.** The most mainstream plan, this form incorporates five Lean and Green Fuelings and one adjusted Lean and Green supper every day.

- **Ideal Weight 4&2&1 Plan.** For the individuals who need more calories or adaptability in food decisions, this arrangement incorporates four Lean and Green Fuelings, two Lean and Green suppers, and one nibble for each day.

- **Ideal Health 3&3 Plan.** Intended for support, this one incorporates three Lean and Green Fuelings and three adjusted Lean and Green dinners every day.

The Lean and Green program gives extra devices to help weight reduction and upkeep, including tips and motivation through instant message, network discussions, week after week bolster calls and an application that permits you to set feast updates and track food admission and action.

The organization likewise gives particular projects to nursing moms, more seasoned grown-ups, adolescents, and individuals with diabetes or gout.

In spite of the fact that Lean and Green offers these particular plans, it's muddled whether this eating routine is alright for individuals with certain ailments. Moreover, young people and breastfeeding moms have extraordinary supplement and calorie needs that may not be met by the Lean and Green diet.

Explanation of How a Holoprotein Regimen Works and Why It Leads to Weight-Loss Results

The Optimal Weight 5&1 Strategy, which requires five fuels a day, is adopted by most dieters. You may select from more than 60 choices, including shakes, soups, bars, biscuits, and pudding, many of which contain a probiotic that the company claims encourage digestive health and high-quality protein. Your sixth regular meal, which you may have at any point, is made up of prepared lean protein, three portions of veggies, and good fats.

You'll collaborate with Lean and Green coaches while on a diet and become a member of a group to support your progress further. When you hit your target weight, it is potentially simpler to move from the diet, and your old behaviors are substituted with new ones. Via its Optimum Fitness 3&3 Plan, the company delivers a specific range of items tailored for weight management.

For people searching for a much more customizable yet higher-calorie diet, Lean and Green also provides the Ideal Weight 4&2&1 Package, which involves four fueling, two Lean and Green portions, and one healthy snack, such as a fruit or a sweet potato portion. The company also promotes special programs for people with asthma, nursing mothers, individuals with gout, the elderly, and teenagers.

Lean and Green diet eating strategies differ somewhat based on how much weight you need to lose and how early you are in the path of weight reduction, although all diets consist of two key elements: Lean and Green Meals and Fueling.

Fueling are Lean and Green 's pre-packaged meals intended to be "nutritively interchangeable food replacements that are carb-controlled and low in fat," with choices varying from bars, cookies, and shakes to more nutritious meals such as Spinach Mac & Cheese with pesto you cook your own, Lean and Green Meals and rely on lean protein, balanced fats, and vegetables that are from lower-carb. Plans differ depending on the amount of regular recommended Lean and Green Meals and Fueling (see below) steadily growing in calories and carbohydrates.

- 5&1 Schedule 1 Lean and Green Meal and 5 Fueling 800 to 1000 Cal.

- 4&2&1 Schedule 2 Lean and Green Meals, 5 Fueling and 1 Nutritious snack 1100−1300 Cal.

- 5&2&1 Schedule 2 Lean and Green Meals, 5 Fueling, and 2 Nutritious Snacks from 1300 to 1500 calories

- 3&3 Schedule 3 Lean and Green Meals and Fueling 1500 to 1800 Cal.

- One fruit or low-fat dairy serving is deemed a nutritious snack.

To encourage weight reduction, Lean and Green depends on intensively reducing calories. Most Fuelings produce about 100−110 calories, which ensures you can eat about 1,000 calories a day on this diet.

How You Will Have to Eat After Doing Lean and Green Diet?

When embarking on any new diet regimen, you may experience some difficulties along the way. Below are the reasons why this diet regimen is considered the easiest to follow among all commercial diet regimens:

- **Eating out can be challenging but still possible:** If you love eating out, you can download Lean and Green's dining out guide. The guide comes with tips on how to navigate buffets, order beverages, and choose condiments. Aside from following the guide, you can also ask the chef to make substitutions for the ingredients used in cooking your food. For instance, you can ask the chef to serve no more than 7 ounces of steak and serve it with steamed broccoli instead of baked potatoes.

- **Opt for lean and green foods that have high fullness index:** Eat foods that contain high protein and fiber content as they can keep you full for longer periods. In fact, many nutrition experts highlight the importance of satiety when it comes to weight loss.

- **You have access to knowledgeable coaches:** If you follow the Lean and Green Diet plan, you have access to knowledgeable coaches and become a part of a community that will give you access to support calls and community events. You also have a standby nutrition support team that can answer your questions.

How Simple Is It to Follow Lean and Green Diet? Is Physical Activity Recommended on the Lean and Green Diet?

Regardless of the plan you choose, you start by having a phone conversation with a coach to help determine which Lean and Green plan to follow, set weight loss goals, and familiarize yourself with the program.

Initial Steps

You're meant to eat 1 meal every 2–3 hours and incorporate 30 minutes of moderate exercise most days of the week.

In total, the Fuelings and meal provide no more than 100 grams of carbs per day.

The program also includes a dining-out guide that explains how to order a Lean and Green meal at your favorite restaurant. Keep in mind that alcohol is strongly discouraged on the 5&1 Plan.

Maintenance Phase

Those who experience sustained success on the program have the option to become trained as an Lean and Green coach.

Exercise and the Lean and Green Diet?

The group suggests 30 minutes of a moderate-intensity exercise similar to walking. Other activities that you can efficiently perform daily is suitable when you are on an Lean and Green diet. However, whatever exercise you decide to follow, make sure you start slowly and gradually increase the time and strength as your body allows. You will always run out of energy if you go overboard on the exercise. The Optimal Weight 5 & 1 package offers particular suggestions.

Comparison with Other Diets. What Do the Experts Say About the Lean and Green Diet?

Comparative Diets

There are a few famous diet plans that are like Lean and Green, yet with key contrasts that may impact whether they are a solid match for your objectives.

SlimFast Diet

At the point when you consider supper substitutions, SlimFast presumably strikes a chord first. While the food and item parts of SlimFast and Lean and Green 's plans are comparative, there are some key contrasts.

SlimFast's variety of dinner substitution items is comparable in nourishment, yet you won't find as much assortment likewise with Lean and Green 's plan.

In any case, a trait of SlimFast is that it offers supper supplanting lines that consent to unique diets, for example, Keto and Diabetic weight-loss.

In the event that you like having worked in social help and training, that is a key element of Lean and Green 's plan that you won't find with a SlimFast diet.

Simple K Diet

Another well-known feast substitution plan is the Special K diet. To follow the fourteen-day "challenge," you'll supplant two dinners per day with Special K grain or another Special K item. At that point, have your standard supper.

The Special K diet is basically a "convenient solution" or "crash diet" and isn't expected for longer-term use.

Lean and Green 's 5&1 plan additionally offers brisk weight loss yet with more assortment than two dinners of oat daily.

With Lean and Green, you can likewise change to the 3 & 3 or 4 & 2 & 1 plans for weight support once you meet your underlying objective.

Whenever the cost is your principal thought, fourteen days' of the Special K diet is unquestionably a less expensive alternative than most diet programs—including Lean and Green 's.

Nutrisystem

Like Lean and Green, Nutrisystem is a supper substitution organization that sends clients pre-made, pre-bundled nourishments that remove the planning and mystery from dinner prep and planning.

In any case, as opposed to Lean and Green 's Fuelings, Nutrisystem's items all the more intently take after ordinary suppers.

Nutrisystem's food decisions, for example, pizza, sandwiches, and macintosh and cheddar are proposed to sub for every one of the three suppers per day.

Recommendations by USDA

The Lean and Green Diet digresses from wellbeing and sustenance rules supported by the United States Department of Agriculture (USDA) in a few regions.

The USDA's Dietary Guidelines for Americans 2015–2020 gauge that a sound grown-up requires 1600 to 3000 calories for every day, contingent upon their movement level.

In spite of the fact that Lean and Green 's 5&1 plan is expected for weight loss, the 800 to 1000 carbohydrate level for each day is an extraordinary decrease from the USDA's suggestion.

One region where Lean and Green goes amiss from USDA suggestions is as far as macronutrients—explicitly, starches.

Lean and Green 's plans allegedly give 80 to 100 grams of sugars every day. As such, about 40% of the diet's everyday calories originate from carbs, though the USDA Dietary Guidelines prescribe a diet that is 45 to 65% sugars.

The USDA additionally accentuates that a smart dieting plan incorporates grains and dairy items, which are not spoken to in Lean and Green 's 5&1 plan.

Why Will Lean and Green Diet Help You in Weight-Loss?

The primary reason why the Lean and Green diet was developed is to help people lose weight and fat by cutting their carbs and calories through portion-controlled snacks and meals.

The 5&1 plan is not going beyond 800–1,000 calories per day for a maximum number of 6 portioned-controlled meals.

Studies of people that have taken this diet plan show that it can be very effective in achieving weight loss than traditional calorie-restricted diets. A 16-week study conducted on 198 people who are obese or have excess weight shows that those who took Lean and Green's 5&1 plan were able to lower their weight significantly as well as their waist circumference and their fat levels. However, those in the control group were not able to achieve such a level of success.

Specifically, the result shows that those that engage in the 5&1 plan were able to shed over 5.7% of their weight, and 28.1% of them were able to lose 10% of their weight. Hence, this diet plan can guarantee a 5-10% weight loss with a lower risk of the type of diabetes and heart disease.

The record has it that those on the 5&1 diet plan and who took part in up to 75% of their coaching sessions can shed twice as much weight as those that participate in fewer coaching sessions. Hence, this shows that if you take the diet plan, the coaching session is crucial as it is one of the determinants for your successful weight loss.

In essence, the Lean and Green diet is a useful tool in losing weight on a short-term basis, which is very obvious since you will be consuming calories that is just about half of the recommended calories for adults.

Some Scientific Research

How much you lose with the Lean and Green diet plans based on factors such as your beginning weight and size, and how much you conform to the schedule, and how healthy you are?

Lean and Green reflects the coach group and lifestyle brand, introduced in 2017. Previous experiments were conducted using the products f another company and not the current Lean and Green goods. Since the Lean and Green goods are a new brand, the old company has told the U.S. Reports that they have the same macronutrient profile and are comparable to theirs as well. Therefore, when testing this diet, we conclude the following findings are essential. There has been no literature conducted directly on the label Lean and Green.

The trials were limited, with several dropouts, as is familiar with most diets. Quick-term, it appears difficult not to lose at least a few pounds; you consume half the calories that other people receive. The study seems to back it up. Long-range views are less optimistic. Look at the details in more depth here: A 2016 research partially funded by this company and reported in the journal Obesity showed that obese people lost 8.8% of their body weight with their drugs and Lean and Green's Style Counseling after 12 weeks, and 12.1% of the body mass if they took phentermine at the same time, a weight-loss medication that may minimize food cravings.

A 2017 company-Sponsored Analysis showed that more than 70% of overweight individuals who earned one-on-one clinical assistance lose more than 5% of the bodyweight after their last appointment (anything between 4 to 24 weeks later).

A research conducted by Johns Hopkins Medicine in 2015 found no credible proof that certain mainstream weight-loss services resulted in long-term weight reduction for humans. The researchers analyzed articles on randomized clinical experiments that lasted for 12 weeks or more. In studies lasting four to six months, participants in a low-calorie diet plan, lose a lot of weight than nonparticipants. But the researchers noticed only one long-term analysis, which at 12 months demonstrated little value to such plans. The researchers also find that the relatively low-calorie systems carried greater chances of injuries, including gallstones.

A 2015 research released in the Annals of Internal Medicine reviewed at 45 similar studies, with generic and patented weight-loss programs. Relatively low-calorie plans, culminated in a weight reduction of 4% better than therapy at four months. But the analysis showed some of this impact lessened after six months of publishing.

A 2015 research in the Diet Journal examined at the charts of 310 overweight and obese clients of this company who adopted the Accomplish Schedule and noticed who those who were on the schedule dropped a total of around 24 pounds by twelve weeks as well as 35 pounds by twenty-four weeks. No matter their age or ethnicity, participants lost more fat instead of lean muscle.

Global research, sponsored and planned by this company and reported in Nutrition Journal in 2010, has randomly allocated 90 obese adults to either the 5&1 regimen or a calorie-restricted plan based on government recommendations. Those in the Lean and Green category had dropped a total of 30 pounds after 16 weeks, relative to the other group 14 pounds. Yet 24 weeks later, the Lean and Green dieters had lost more than 10 pounds as dieters steadily upped their calories, while the others had placed back on only 2 pounds. The Lean and Green group at week 40 had fewer body fat and much more lean muscle than at the outset but did not substantially outperform the controlled experiment. Nearly half of the Lean and Green party and much more than half of its control community had ended up dropping out.

A company's Funded Survey of 119 obese or overweight Type 2 diabetics, reported in the Diabetes Educator (2008), randomly allocated dietitians to a Lean and Green diabetic regimen or a diet focused on American Diabetes Association guidelines. After 34 weeks, the Lean and Green party had lost 10 1/2 pounds but had recovered all but 3 pounds after 86 weeks. At 34 weeks, the diabetics on the ADA-based diet dropped a total of 3 pounds; at 86 weeks, they'd won it all back plus a pound. The rate of dropout was almost 80%.

In a 2008 company's Funded Study released in the journal Eating and Weight Problems, researchers analyzed the patient history of 324 overweight or obese Lean and Green dietitians who were both taking a prescription appetite suppressant. On average, the patients weighed 21 pounds at 12 weeks, 26 1/2 pounds at 24 weeks, and 27 pounds at 52 weeks.

Additionally, during all three tests, about 80% of them had lost at least 5% of their original weight. That's not terrible—dropping only 5 or 10% of your current weight can help stave off specific ailments if you're overweight. These statistics, though, come with a set of asterisks. Firstly, these are focused on completers, including people who completed the 52-week regimen and became more inclined to lose weight. (Weight reduction was also significant but less severe in an investigation that compensated for dropouts.) Second, a summary of medical reports holds less weight than a sample of a test group. Finally, the weight reduction was not substantially different in a study where researchers separated dieters into categories of regular Lean and Green consumers (those who registered to drink at least two shakes a day at each check-in) and unreliable ones (the rest).

A 2013 research in the International Journal of Obesity examined 120 men and women aged 19 to 65, half of which utilized Lean and Green products, and the other half were merely reducing calories. Researchers noticed that people on the lean and Green diet lost a total of 16 1/2 pounds over 26 weeks, contrasted with the placebo group, which lost 8 pounds.

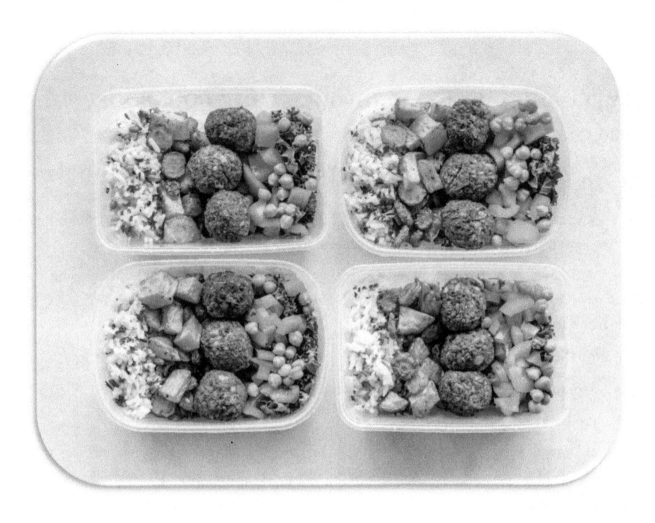

SIMPLE AND EASY LEAN AND GREEN DIET COOKBOOK
Meal Planner + Shopping List

Meal planning becomes simple in the 5&1 plan when you know the nutritional parameters of a Lean and Green meal according to your lean protein options, a Lean & Green meal contains 5 to 7 ounces of prepared lean protein with three portions of vegetables that are not starchy, and up to two portions of healthy fats.

Savor your Lean & Green meal—whenever it fits best on your timetable, at any time of day. If you're eating out or monitoring your consumption, use the Lean & Green Meal Nutritional Criteria given below to direct your choices better:

Nutritional Criteria of L&G Meal Calories

- 250-400 Calories Carbs ≤ 20 g of total carbohydrate (ideally < 15 g).

- Protein >= 25 g Fat 10–20 g.

The three key components of each Lean and Green meal are Protein, Good Fats, and Carbohydrates.

The list of ingredients you would need to make a balanced meal and shop according to your meal schedule is provided below.

Protein is classified into the lean, leaner, and leanest types. Purchase groceries according to recipes of your liking and recipe them to your taste.

Leanest: Pick a 7-oz. The cooked part, which has 0-4 g of net fat, then includes 2 healthy fat servings.

- Fish: cod, haddock, flounder, rough orange, tilapia, grouper, haddock, Mahi Mahi, wild catfish, tuna canned in water).

- Shellfish: scallops, crab, lobster, shrimp.

- Game meat: buffalo, deer, elk turkey (Ground).

- Other meat: around 98% lean.

- Meatless choices: 14 whites of eggs 2 cups of liquid egg white or liquid egg replacement 5 oz. seitan 1½ cups or 2 oz. of 1% cottage cheese 12 ounces. of Non-fat (0%) regular Greek yogurt (approximately 15 g carb per 12 ounces).

Leaner: Pick a 6 oz. The part cooked, which has 5–9 g of net fat and includes 1 portion of Healthy Fat.

- Fish species: swordfish, halibut, trout, white meat.

- Chicken breast skin-free turkey (Ground).

- Other poultry: 95%–97% lean meat.

- Turkey: light poultry.

- Meatless choices: Two entire eggs or four egg whites Two entire eggs and one cup of liquid egg replacer 1 ½ cups or 12 oz. or 2% cottage cheese 12 ounces. Low fat (2%) regular Greek yogurt (approximately 15 g carb per 12 ounces).

Lean: Pick a part of 5 oz. Cooked with 10g-20 g net fat-no extra portion of healthy fat.

- Fish: tuna (bluefin steak), salmon, catfish farmed, herring, mackerel.

- Lean beef: roasted, ground, steak.

- Lamb pork fillet or Porkchop turkey (Ground).

- Other poultry: 85%-94% leaner meat.

- Turkey or chicken: dark meat.

- Meatless choices: 15 ounces. Extra-firm or firm (bean curd) tofu Three eggs whole (up to 2 days a week) 4 ounces. part-skim cheese or Reduced-fat (3-6g fat per ounce) (1 cup shredded) 8 ounces. (1 cup) ricotta part-skim cheese (2-3 g of fat per ounce.) 5-ounce.

Tempe Healthy Amounts of Fat

There can be around 5 g of fat and less than 5 g of carb in a portion of healthy fat. Include 0–2 Healthy Fat Portions daily Depending on your options for lean: 1 tsp of oil (any sort), 1 tbsp of normal, low-carb dressing for the salad 2 tbsp. lowered-fat, low-carb dressing for the salad 5–10 green or black olives 1 ½ ounce. Avocado ⅓ ounce. Simple nuts, such as almonds, pistachios, or peanuts 1 tbsp. of simple seeds, such as sesame, flax, chia, or seeds of pumpkin, ½ tbsp. regular margarine, butter, or mayonnaise.

Green & Lean Meal: The "Greens"

Greens make up a substantial proportion of the carbohydrates eaten in the 5&1 diet.

Pick three servings from our green choices collection for each of your meals (Lean & Green). We've sorted the choices for vegetables into the amounts of lower, medium, and higher carb levels. Every one of them is acceptable on the Optimum Weight 5 & 1 meal plan; the list assists you to make responsible choices on food.

From the Green Choice List, pick 3 servings: 1 serving = ½ cup (except where specified) of vegetables with around 25 calories and around 5 g of carbohydrates.

- **Low Carb:** 1 cup: endive, green leaf lettuce, Butterhead, romaine, iceberg, collard (fresh/raw), spinach (fresh/raw), mustard greens, watercress, bok choy (raw), spring mix ½ cup: cucumbers, radishes, white mushrooms, sprouts (Mung bean, alfalfa), turnip greens, celery, arugula, escarole, Swiss chard (raw), jalapeño (raw), bok choy (cooked), nopales.

- **Moderate Carb:** ½ cup: cabbage, eggplant, cauliflower, fennel bulb, asparagus, Mushrooms, Kale, portabella, summer squash (scallop or zucchini) cooked spinach.

- **Higher Carb:** ½ cup: red cabbage, squash, collard, chayote squash(cooked) mustard greens, green or wax beans, broccoli, kabocha squash, (cooked) leeks, Kohlrabi, okra, (any color) peppers, scallions (raw), (crookneck or straightneck) summer squash, Turnips, Tomatoes, Spaghetti Squash, Palm Cores, Jicama, Swiss (cooked) chard.

Sample Meal Plan Sample

The meal plan of the Optimal 5&1 program is very easy and simple to follow.

The fuelings are readily available in pre-packaged and ready to eat form.

The only prep you need is for a Lean and Green meal, which is also made easy for you by providing you with easy recipes and a grocery list. A sample meal plan is provided to help you understand the simplicity of this weight-loss program.

A Day in the Optimal 5&1 Plan Fueling

- 1 ex: Caramel Mocha Shake Fueling.

- 2 ex: Creamy Double Crisp Peanut Butter Bar Fueling.

- 3 ex: Roasted Creamy Garlic Smashed Potatoes Fueling.

- 4 ex: Cinnamon Sugary Sticks Fueling.

- 5 ex: Chewy Dewy Chocolate Chip Biscuit.

- Lean & Green Meal (your favorite recipe from this book).

- Water Intake (check off how many glasses of water you have each day) = 8 oz.

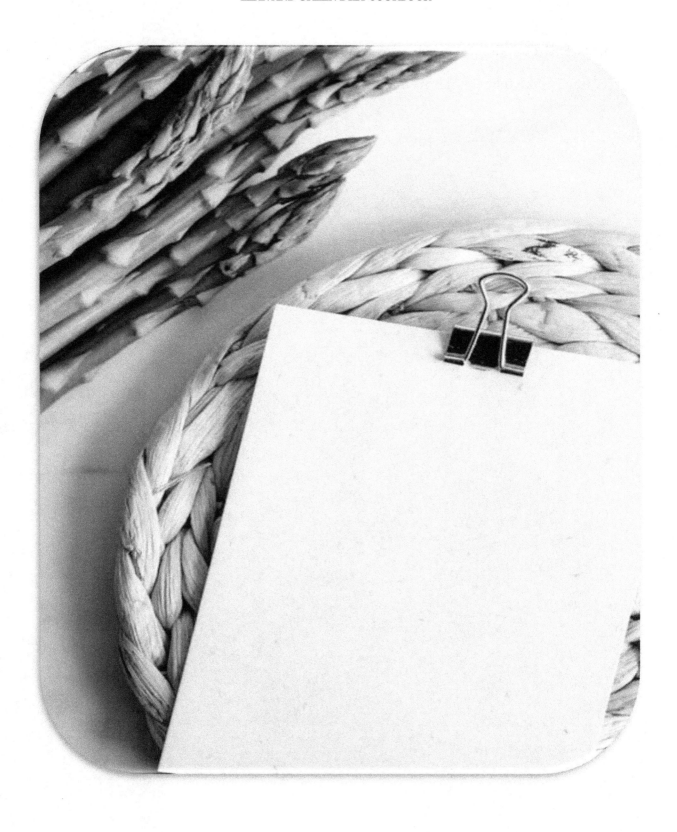

RECOMMENDED COOKING METHODS

Slow cookers are safe and easy to use. It's as simple as preparing ingredients, securing the lid, turning on the machine, and setting the timer. Once you've done all those necessary steps, then you're good to go, literally.

Gone are the days when you have to watch over the whole process of cooking or stir the contents of the pot often. Using a slow cooker lets you leave it overnight, so you can warm the dish the next day, or leave it while you go to work during the day, so it will be ready when you get home. You can also prepare large volumes of dishes during the weekend sans slaving hours in the kitchen.

The slow cooker also uses approximately 15 to 30 watts per hour.

When using the slow cooker for the first time, it is important to take note of the following:

1. **Different Machines Have Different Setting**

Models vary greatly. Some slow cooker models do not have buttons or settings. All you have to do is plug it and leave your dish to cook on its own. These machines are usually pre-set on medium heat. Therefore, if you are using this kind of model, make sure that you lessen the cooking time for dishes recommended on low heat and then extend the cooking time for recipes recommended on high heat setting.

If the "Warm" function is available. Always ensure that you automatically shift to "Warm Mode." But regardless of your slow cooker has this function or not, your dish remains warm for up to 2 hours after cooking time.

2. **All Ingredients Must Be Thawed Well Before Cooking**

If you are using frozen veggies or meat, make sure to put them at the lower part of the fridge to drain all liquids before placing them inside the slow cooker. Doing so will allow the ingredient/s to keep heat constant and prevent food from retaining too much moisture.

3. **Add Plenty of Liquids**

This is another vital rule when you are slow cooking. You would need to fill the crockpot at least three-quarters up to prevent ingredients from sticking to the bottom of the pan. This will also prevent liquids from boiling over, which could potentially damage the machine. If the dishes have sauces, this is, of course, an exception. Make sure to adjust the volume of the liquid accordingly.

4. Take note of ingredients that are only meant to be added one hour or half an hour at the end of the cooking cycle time or oftentimes, before serving the dish

There are also food items that only require residual heat to cook through.

Knowing about this will help prevent your food from losing texture, flavor, color, and even avoid boiling over. Also, when dealing with seafood, it is best that you only add them at the last hour or stage of cooking, or else, you'll end up serving soggy fish or dried up shellfish.

5. Some Dishes Would Require Pre-Cooking

Why is this necessary, you might ask? This is because food tastes a lot better when lightly seared or browned first. Some of them include chicken, pork, and beef.

The practice of browning meat helps enhance the depth of flavor, which means you can get more flavor out of the ingredients instead of relying on seasonings to do their job of flavoring the dish. And since this eBook is meant for people with kidney problems, this step is of greater importance, especially since you will be taking out salt off the list of seasonings.

You will also notice that some recipes require the sautéing of aromatics such as onion, garlic, and ginger in a skillet before slow cooking. This is another vital step in making your dishes more flavorful. Although some slow cooker models have a "Saute" function, it is still recommended that you do the sautéing in a separate skillet so you will have control over the heat.

Sautéing in a separate pan will also help you prepare for other ingredients of the recipes that would require deglazing or even those garnishes that you put on top of the dish just before serving. Some of the examples include toasted garlic, bacon bits, or even eggs, etc.

6. Let Your Meals Cook Uninterrupted

When cooking, most people have the habit of removing the lid, stirring ingredients, and visually checking on the food from time to time. If you are going to use a slow cooker, this will not be necessary at all. Let your food be cooked undisturbed, or at least for the first 2−4 hours of cooking time before stirring.

When you make use of the slow cooker, remember to secure the lid and avoid lifting it as this may cause the temperature to drop drastically, or worse, cause injuries and accidents. If you can't stop yourself from virtually checking what you're cooking from time to time, purchase a slow cooker that has glass lids where you can easily peer into.

7. Season Your Meals Before Serving

There are some food items such as bone-in beef, ham knuckles, potatoes, carrots, and sweet potatoes that can release or retain more flavor after cooking for a longer period.

On the other hand, you also have to be mindful of food items that tend to lose their flavor and taste after they are cooked for more than 20 minutes. Some of them include seafood, shellfish, lemon, fish, lime, and tamarinds.

Finally, seasoning before serving your cooked meals will help you gauge the taste of the food. Seasoning before cooking only gives you more reason to add more flavorings and seasonings in the process. So to ensure that you don't end up with overly salty food, season after you have turned off the slow cooker or just before serving meals.

8. A Squeeze of Lemon or Lime Will Do the Trick for Leftover Food

Some say that slow-cooked meals are at their best taste a day or two in the freezer. To keep your dishes tastier when you reheat them, add a few drops of lime or lemon to help stimulate the taste. For sweet meals, adding a pinch of sugar will make it taste better after reheating. For spicy food, adding minced chilies will make the dish more flavorful and hot.

9. Always Garnish Your Food. Garnish Your Dishes with Fresh Herbs, Spices, Fruits or Vegetables.

When you use the slow cooker, there are some food items or ingredients that turn dull and become two shades darker. So to make them at least pleasing to the eyes, always remember to garnish with freshly chopped herbs and spices, fruits, vegetables, cheese, and even nuts. This will help make the dishes more enticing to eat and visually appealing. Try garnishing with vibrantly colored spices such as Spanish paprika and fresh chilies, among others.

You can also try serving your dish with colorful side dishes such as carrots, corn, peas, lettuce, or lemon wedges.

10. When It Comes to Washing and Cleaning the Slow Cooker, Make Sure to Allow the Machine to Cool Down at Room Temperature Before Washing Completely

This is particularly helpful in prolonging the life of your machine. Immediately washing it with cold water will cause the machine to crack and the metal to warp. The best time to wash the slow cooker is at least 2 hours after. Should some food items stick to the bottom of the crockpot, wash it with warm water with drops of dishwashing solution. Set aside before drying and storing.

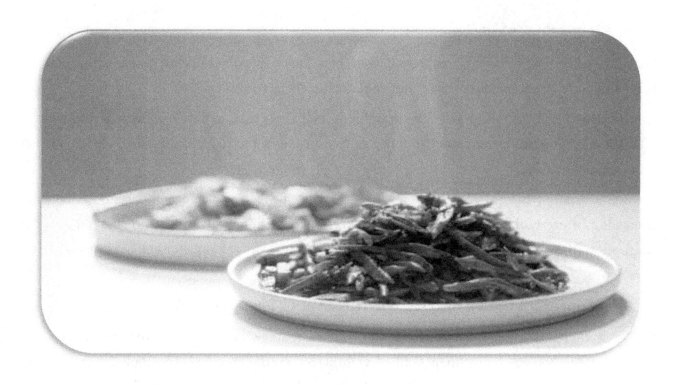

TRICKS TO ELIMINATE THE FOOD SCALE

When you're dining, maintain the power of portion sizes. If you have a supersize amount, ask for a to-go bag as the meal is brought to your table and bring half of the meal in for tomorrow instantly. Share aperitifs, entrees, and treats. Half the dish represents half the calories. Place your utensils in between the bites to help slow your eating down. Emphasis on talk and companionship rather than the meal. When you have done consuming a balanced amount, make your plate clean.

Chinese Food

Steamed lean protein and veggies are as good as possible, but such sauces are another matter. If you obey these recommendations, staying safe at Chinese restaurants could be a "wok in the park":

- Select vegetable-rich dishes and ask for additional vegetables (especially in beef broccoli, green beans, or mushrooms with chicken).

- Still inquire for side sauce. It is the sauces that are usually very heavy in salt and carbohydrates.

- Order the preparation of dishes without nuts or seeds

- Question about the quality and practice of things you may be confused about, such as:

  o Chinese or mix vegetables

  o Special sauces

  o Soups (egg white, ginger, etc.)

- Question if products are prepared with sugar, maize starch, or flour coating and question for stir-fried or steamed meat and vegetables to be "pure."

- Using soy sauce of low sodium content.

- Use chopsticks to minimize the number of sauces you consume to help slow down your diet.

- Evite products that are defined as crispy, lightly browned, or sweet-and-sour, as they are typically deep-fried.

- In repair, settle for steamed rice instead of fried rice, or inquire to add brown rice or, at most, a side of extra veggies.

When you are on a weight losing part of the 5&1 Plan:

- "Diet" or "balanced" dishes: These are usually the best alternatives for dining in Chinese restaurants; such dishes are generally steamed and can be cooked without adding oil, cornstarch, sugar, MSG, or salt. Make sure to inquire about unique topics and methods for the training.

  Pick these dishes:

  o Mixed vegetable chicken.

  o Mixed vegetable shrimp.

  o Mixed veggies.

  o Simple broccoli.

  o Veggies like green beans, broccoli, mushrooms, having lean protein such as poultry, shrimp, scallop, beef, or tofu.

- Certain Lean & Green Meal friendly food items:

  o Vegetables and lean meat shish kebabs.

  o Moo Goo Gai Pan: Stir-fried poultry and (usually) mushrooms.

  o Szechuan prawns, poultry, shrimps, beef, or lean meat.

  o Curry shrimps, squid, lamb, etc.

  o Sha Cha dishes: sauce or paste is often referred to as "Chinese barbecue sauce" and is usually produced from garlic, soya oil, chilis, brilliant fish, and dried shrimps. It has a savory, often hot, taste, fine with beef or chicken.

  o Lobster sauce shrimp.

  o Grilled meat, fish, or (lean) steamed vegetable beef.

When you're in the Weight-Maintenance Phase: Pick each of the above products (continuing to look at portion sizes and salt levels, as these can be large when it relates to Chinese food) and take into account the following recommendations:

- Consider broth-based soups: wonton, egg drop, or hot & sour.

- Instead of an egg roll, pick a spring roll.

- Order steamed green dumplings instead of fried or pork dumplings. (These also contain many calories but are a better substitute to an egg roll while wanting fried something.)

- Swap meals: Order fewer meals than people in the restaurant; choose at least one vegetarian choice, like:

  o Steamed broccoli, green beans, or mixed vegetables.

  o "Buddha's Joy."

  o Ma Po (Hunan) tofu.

  o Mu Shu beef, chicken, tofu, or pork.

Fast Food

Fast food is all over the place; inexpensive and easy. Yet much of it still has high fat, sugar, and calories portion. To eat a quick snack without losing your healthier weight, obey these basic guidelines:

- Be mindful that, in terms of calories, fat, and calcium, not all nutritious salads and entrees are delicious.

- Evite some fried food as it appears to be filled with saturated "bad" fat.

- Stop consuming soft drinks or sweetened beverages containing high fructose corn syrup (although free refills are tempting).

- Do not "super-scale" or "max the worth" of your meal. When it endangers your fitness plans by consuming three or four times more than you can consume, it is not a discount.

- Order meals for infants, which are smaller.

- Don't order the meals in combination. While they can be handy, they add more calories to your diet; stick with individual products.

When you are on a Weight-Losing Part of the 5&1 Plan:

- Enjoy the beef without the crust for the chicken sandwiches or hamburgers.

- Garnish with grilled meat, not fried or breaded (no poultry or nuggets).

- Inquire for all seasonings, dressings, and side sauces.

When you're in the Weight-Maintenance Phase:

- Skip the bacon or butter. Ask for a little bit on the side if you're missing these additions.

- When you choose anything delicious, avoid the cookies and ice cream and just select a fruit portion.

- Miss mayonnaise or "special sauces" full of calories, fat, and even sugar. The fat and calories are smaller than ketchup, vinegar, pickles, and onions.

- Create an open-faced sandwich with the top burger bun or lunch roll cut, meaning you have less processed white flour.

Greek Food

Greek cuisine is overflowing with new herbs, pork, chicken, and olive oil, ensuring there are loads of nutrient-filled, balanced food options. You will reap the advantages here while reducing unnecessary calories and fats:

- To prevent excess salt and fat, restrict the nuts and feta cheese.

- Fix your dishes with light cuts of beef, lamb, and seafood.

- Bear in mind that a bit of olive oil makes a huge difference, so just drizzle sufficiently to moisturize your stuff.

When You Are on a Weight-Losing Part of the 5&1 Plan:

- Olive oil is a balanced, monounsaturated "good" fat but does not surpass your safe daytime fat serving(s). Ask to cook your meal with little to no gasoline, to call for it on the floor.

- Evite typical béchamel sauces rich in milk or honey and butter.

- Evite the hummus (a standard Greek chickpea dip), which is rich in carbohydrates. Try:

  - **Greek salad:** miss the feta cheese, and ask for olives and sauce on the table. One good fat is 5 medium olives.

- o **Greek frittata (omelet):** miss the cheese and the potatoes and move the seasonings and olives on the side.
- o **Kebab:** Lean vegetarian kebab beef. Replace with a little bowl the rice or pasta.

When you're in the Weight-Maintenance Phase:

- Add lemon juice rather than using typical cream sauces on your vegetables, meat, and fish.

- As a dessert, prefer fresh fruit.

- When you splurge on a higher-fat inlet, grab a low-fat side salad, like lettuce, to go along.

- Ask for low-fat Greek yogurt as a supplement for regular Greek yogurt, which is heavy in fat if necessary.

Indian Food

New vegetables and spices with aromas prevail in Indian cuisine. Here is how to appreciate the subcontinent's unique flavors while keeping on board with the Lean and Green App:

- Avoid foods that contain ghee, clarified with butter.

- Inquire about your nut-free bowl, as they have several Indian dishes.

- Inquire about side sauces.

- Resist malai ingredients, meaning milk and makhani, made from butter.

- Exclude "crispy" or "golden" fried dishes in the label.

- Stop soups or coconut dishes that are rich in fat.

When you are on a Weight-Losing Part of the 5&1 Plan:

- Consider the given Lean & Green Meal compatible dishes:
  - o **Sabzi, saag,** or bharta: common terminology for cooked veggies.
  - o **Chicken tikka:** bits of skinless or boneless chicken marinated using spices.
  - o **Kebab:** skewered vegetables or meat.
  - o **Keema:** slimming meat dish.
- Also, ask for the vegetables and the meat to be prepared with little or no oil.

When you're in the Weight-Maintenance Phase: Usually, dishes are followed by a slice of bread and a rice serving. Avoid the rice as your bread choice, and also ask for roti. Roti is usually made of wheat grain instead of white flour.

Italian Food

Though tasty and famous, Italian food will test your imagination when you eat healthy, with its bread, pasta, creamy sauces, or cheeses (you can drink wine), but it's not impossible.

Take some tips:

- Remind your server not to deliver bread to the table to prevent any temptations. Most Italian breads are nutritionally deficient, strong in carbohydrates, and rich in calories.

- Stay away from casseroles, kinds of pasta (particularly cheese-packed), and cream-based sauces loaded with fat.

- Skip grain or seed dishes to minimize calories and fat.

- Do not apply salt to your meal because the boiling water and sauces are typically highly salted.

- Fatty and jam-packed with fat and calories; avoid Italian cakes and pastries.

- Skip cheese and croutons on salads.

- Select plates that are high in vegetables.

- Prefer fried, broiled, or grilled meat or seafood, and keep away from breaded options, sliced, or served in some form of sauce.

- Select side sauce. Sauces appear to add a ton of extra calories, carbs, fat, and sodium, particularly Marsala, pesto, Alfredo, Bolognese, marinara, as well as vodka sauce.

- Pick an entry section of an appetizer or side part, along with a salad.

- Pick a meal to share with a buddy, or call for a to-go box before you start dining to dine adequately.

- When buying a meal, select sauce on the table.

- If you are in the repair process and crave sugar, stick to Italian ice cream, biscotti, or condensed milk cappuccino, which is less calorie and fat.

Remember: Higher carbohydrate products such as starchy vegetables (such as potatoes), pasta, beans, bread, and rice are not prescribed during the Lean and Green Program's weight-loss process.

When you are on a Weight-Losing Part of the 5&1 Plan:

- Inquire for meat, pork, scallop, or tuna from your table, and do not have any pasta.

- Appreciate onions, lettuce, mushrooms, berries, asparagus, and broccoli.

- Order meats that have no side covering and gravy.

- Consider salads with grilled tuna, scallops, chicken, or other healthy protein, and no croutons or cheese.

When you're in the Weight-Maintenance Phase:

- Order your whole wheat pizza or pasta, or whole wheat dough, if appropriate.

- Select low-fat cheeses and pasta or pie toppings.

- No to any substitute cheese choices.

- Look for additional spices or herbs to enhance color.

- Pour in soups made from water, such as Italian wedding soup or minestrone.

Mexican Food

While each restaurant is distinct, many U.S. Mexican restaurants rely on Tex-Mex type foods served with cheese, sour cream, and lard, or fried in oil. Through adopting these rules, you will experience a fiesta with tasty, balanced tastes:

- Remind your server not to carry tortilla chips to the table to survive any snacking urges.

- Order plates full of healthy vegetables and protein.

- Servings of Mexican food at the restaurant can be massive. Share lunch with a mate, or avoid eating after consuming the right quantity of food and saving the remainder for tomorrow in a to-go refrigerator.

Remember: Higher carbohydrate foods, such as starchy vegetables (such as corn), rice, beans, tortillas, or chips, are not suggested during the Lean and Green Program weight-loss process.

When you are on a Weight-Losing Part of the 5&1 Plan: Suggestions of Mexican restaurant meals that are Lean & Green Meal compliant:

- Taco salad: order without guacamole, sour cream, cheese, or fried tortilla dish, either with side dressing.

- Meat or veggie fajitas, consumed without cheese, tortillas, guacamole, or sour cream.

- Some grilled beef, chicken, or seafood without cheese, tortilla shells, guacamole, or sour cream.

- Please require that your order be delivered with no butter or lard included.

When you're in the Weight-Maintenance Phase:

- To minimize fat and calories, order your meal without cheese and sour cream (or ask for that at the side).

- For a fiery pop, savor your meal with a Pico de Gallo, new salsa, or jalapeños.

- Stop fried beans since they are usually produced with lard and extra salt. Choose simple black or red or drunken beans instead.

- Welcome soft seasoning to remove sodium.

- Select corn tortillas that could be loaded with saturated fats instead of wheat ones.

- In balance, including the guacamole. While guacamole is full of healthy fats, calories are also loaded on it.

- Stop fried quesadillas, filled with meat, calories, and fat.

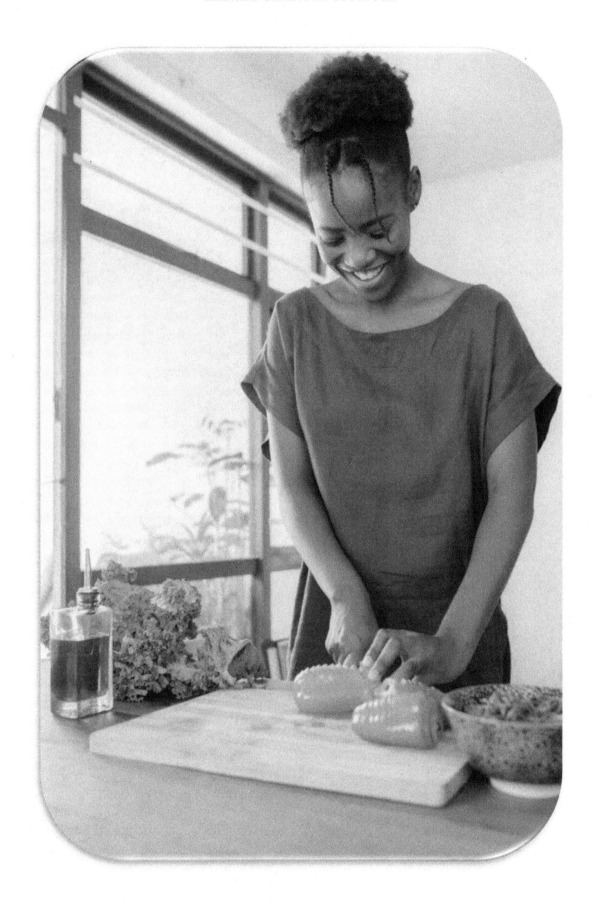

SMOOTHIES AND BREAKFASTS

• Chocolate Sweet Potato Pudding

Preparation Time: 5 minutes

Cooking Time: 2 minutes

Servings: 1

INGREDIENTS:

- 2 well-cooked sweet potatoes
- 2 tablespoons cocoa powder
- 2 tablespoons maple syrup
- ¼ cups plant-based milk (for example, almond milk)
- ¼ tablespoons salt
- ¼ tablespoons vanilla extract

DIRECTIONS:

1. Inside the food processor, put all the ingredients.
2. Blend thoroughly for about 30 seconds to 1 minute. Voilà!

NUTRITION :

- Calories: 200
- Fat: 1.5 g
- Carbohydrates: 23.4 g
- Fiber: 1.3 g

• Peanut Butter and Protein Pancake

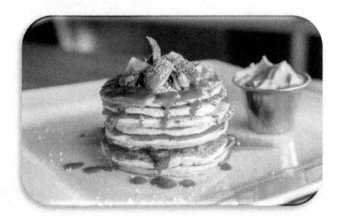

Preparation Time: 10 minutes

Cooking Time: 15 minutes

Servings: 1

INGREDIENTS:

- ½ cup oat flour
- ½ cup gluten-free chocolate pancake mix
- ½ cup almond milk
- 1 egg
- 1 tablespoon coconut water
- 1 tablespoon peanut butter
- Fresh fruits slices

DIRECTIONS:

1. Preheat a saucepan to medium heat.
2. Mix the flour and the pancake; mix in a mixing bowl.
3. Mix the almond milk and eggs with coconut water in another bowl.
4. Mix the dry and wet ingredients thoroughly to form a delicate batter.
5. Spray the preheated saucepan with some coconut oil.
6. Put the batter into the saucepan with a measuring cup and allow it to cook for a few minutes.
7. Allow to cool and top with peanut butter and fresh fruit slices.

NUTRITION

- Calories: 380
- Protein: 22 g
- Carbohydrates: 16 g

• Zucchini Frittata

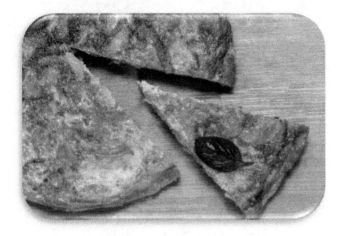

Preparation Time: 20 minutes

Cooking Time: 20 minutes

Servings: 1

INGREDIENTS:

- 2 large zucchinis
- 1½ teaspoon salt
- 2 eggs
- ½ cup chopped green onions
- 1 cup flour
- ½ teaspoon black pepper
- 1 teaspoon baking powder
- 2 tablespoons oil

DIRECTIONS:

1. Wash the two zucchinis.
2. Cut off the zucchinis on its ends and grate them in a large mixing bowl.
3. Stir in 1 teaspoon of salt and set aside for about 10 minutes (The salt helps to draw out the water from the zucchinis).
4. Squeeze dry the grated zucchinis to remove as much water as possible.
5. Then followed by the two whole eggs and the chopped green onions.
6. In a bowl, mix a cup of flour, ½ teaspoon of salt, ½ teaspoon of black pepper, and one teaspoon of baking powder.
7. Next, pour the contents of the smaller bowl into those of the larger bowl containing the grated zucchinis.
8. Stir them all together and make sure they are well mixed.
9. Preheat a saucepan to medium temperature and add two tablespoons of oil.
10. Add the zucchini mixture a heaping tablespoonful at a time.
11. Sauté the mixture for about 4 minutes on each side to achieve a golden-brown color.
12. Add more oil to the pan if needed.
13. Serve and enjoy!

NUTRITION:

- Calories: 200
- Protein: 7 g
- Carbohydrates: 4 g
- Fat: 3.5 g

Tex-Mex Tofu Breakfast Tacos

Preparation Time: 10 minutes

Cooking Time: 15 minutes

Servings: 1

INGREDIENTS:

- 8 oz. firm tofu
- 1 cup well-cooked black bean
- 1/4 red onion
- 1 cup fresh coriander
- 1 ripe avocado
- 1/2 cup salsa
- 1 medium-sized lime
- 5 whole corn tortillas
- 1/2 teaspoon garlic powder
- 1/2 teaspoon chili powder
- 1/8 teaspoon of sea salt
- 1 tablespoon salsa
- 1 tablespoon water

DIRECTIONS:

1. Dice the red onions, avocados, coriander, and keep them in separate bowls.
2. Also, slice the limes and keep them in individual bowls.
3. In a clean towel. Wrap the tofu and place under a cast-iron skillet.
4. In the meantime, heat a saucepan to medium heat.
5. Cook the black beans in the saucepan, add a little amount of salt, cumin, and chili powder.
6. Then decrease the heat to a low simmer and set aside.
7. Add the tofu spices and salsa into a bowl, then add some water and set aside.
8. Heat another skillet to medium heat.
9. Pour some oil into the skillet, and then crumble the tofu into it.
10. Stir-fry for about 5 minutes until the tofu begins to brown.
11. Add some seasoning and continue to cook for about 5 to 10 minutes, and then set aside.
12. Heat the tortillas in the oven to 250°F.
13. Top the tortillas with tofu scramble, avocado, salsa, coriander, black beans, and lime juice.
14. Serve immediately.

NUTRITION:

- Calories: 350
- Fat: 6.5 g
- Carbohydrates: 23.6 g
- Protein: 21.5 g

• Mocha Oatmeal

Preparation Time: 5 minutes

Cooking Time: 10 minutes

Servings: 1

INGREDIENTS:

- 1 banana
- ½ cup oats
- 1 cup coffee
- ¼ teaspoon salt
- 1 teaspoon walnut
- ½ teaspoon cacao powder
- 1 cup milk
- Honey

DIRECTIONS:

1. Preheat a saucepan to medium heat.
2. Put the oats in a saucepan.
3. Slice the banana, mash them, and add them to the oats.
4. Add coffee, walnuts, cacao powder, and salt.
5. Stir, and you may want to wait for it to simmer, practically until the mixture becomes sticky inconsistency.
6. Serve in a bowl and add milk and honey as desired.
7. Enjoy!

NUTRITION:

- Calories: 400
- Carbohydrates: 51 g
- Fats: 5 g
- Fiber: 8 g

- **Black and Blueberry Protein Smoothie**

Preparation Time: 5 minutes

Cooking Time: 0 minutes

Servings: 1

INGREDIENTS:

- 1 cup sugar-free coconut milk (or any other plant-based milk of your choice).

- 1 scoop vanilla or natural protein powder.

- 6 oz. fat-free vanilla Greek yogurt.

- 2 tablespoons of milled flaxseed.

- 1 cup berries (black or blue).

- 1 cup ice.

DIRECTIONS:

1. In the food processor, place all the ingredients.

2. Blend until smooth.

3. Pour into a cup and enjoy.

NUTRITION:

- Calories: 360

- Fats: 1.5 g

- Protein: 49 g

- Carbohydrates: 40 g

- **Shake Cake Fueling**

Preparation Time: 5 minutes

Cooking Time: 0 minutes

Servings: 1

INGREDIENTS:

- 1 packet shakes
- ¼ teaspoon baking powder
- 2 tablespoons eggbeaters or egg whites
- 2 tablespoons water
- Other options that are not compulsory include sweetener, reduced-fat cream cheese, ketchup

DIRECTIONS:

1. Begin by preheating the oven.
2. Mix all the ingredients. Begin with the dry ingredients first before adding the wet ingredients.
3. After the mixture/batter is ready, pour gently into muffin cups.
4. Inside the oven, place, and bake for about 16–18minutes or until it is baked and ready. Allow it to cool completely.
5. Add additional toppings of your choice and ensure your delicious shake cake is refreshing.

NUTRITION:

- Calories: 896
- Fat: 37 g
- Carbohydrate: 115 g
- Protein: 34 g

- **Cauliflower Crust Pizza**

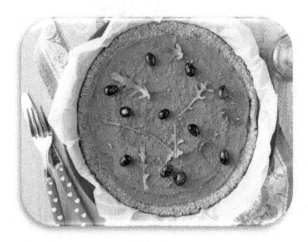

Preparation Time: 15 minutes

Cooking Time: 30 minutes

Servings: 1

INGREDIENTS:

- 1/4 cauliflower (it should be cut into smaller portions)
- 1/16 grated parmesan cheese
- 1/2 egg
- ½ teaspoon Italian seasoning
- 1/16 teaspoon kosher salt
- 1 cups freshly grated mozzarella
- 1/4 cup spicy pizza sauce
- Basil leaves, for garnishing

DIRECTIONS:

1. Begin by preheating your oven while using the parchment paper to rim the baking sheet.

2. Process the cauliflower into a fine powder, and then transfer to a bowl before putting it into the microwave. Leave for about 5–6 minutes to get it soft.

3. Transfer the microwaved cauliflower to a clean and dry kitchen towel. Leave it to cool.

4. When cold, use the kitchen towel to wrap the cauliflower and then get rid of all the moisture by wringing the towel. Continue squeezing until the water is gone completely.

5. Put the cauliflower, Italian seasoning, parmesan, egg, salt, and mozzarella (1 cup). Stir very well until well combined.

6. Transfer the combined mixture to the baking sheet previously prepared, pressing it into a 10-inch round shape.

7. Wait for it to bake until it becomes golden in color.

8. Take the baked crust out of the oven and use the spicy pizza sauce and mozzarella (the leftover 1 cup) to top it. Put it again inside the oven for 10 more minutes until the cheese melts and looks bubbly.

9. Garnish using fresh basil leaves. You can also enjoy this with salad.

NUTRITION:

- Calories: 230
- Fat: 8 g
- Carbohydrate: 28 g
- Protein: 6 g

- **Zucchini Fritters**

Preparation Time: 5 minutes

Cooking Time: 15 minutes

Servings: 1

INGREDIENTS:

- 1/4 pound grated zucchini
- 1/4 teaspoon salt
- 1/16 cup grated parmesan
- 1/16 cup flour
- 1/2 cloves minced garlic
- 1/2 tablespoon olive oil
- 1/4 large egg
- Newly ground black pepper and kosher salt to taste

DIRECTIONS:

1. Put the grated zucchini into a colander over the sink.

2. Add your salt and toss it to mix properly, then leave it to settle for about 10 minutes.

3. Next, use a clean cheesecloth to drain the zucchini completely.

4. Combine drained zucchini, parmesan, garlic, flour, and the beaten egg in a large bowl, mix, and season with pepper and salt.

5. Then, pour the olive oil into a skillet applying medium-high heat.

6. Use a tablespoon to scoop batter for each fritter, put in the oil, and flatten using a spatula.

7. Allow to cook until the underside is richly golden brown, then flip over to the other side and cook.

8. Your delicious zucchini fritters are ready to be served.

NUTRITION:

- Calories: 105.1
- Fat: 2.8 g
- Carbohydrate: 15.8 g
- Protein: 6 g

- **Lean and Green Pizza Hack**

Preparation Time: 5 minutes

Cooking Time: 20 minutes

Servings: 1

INGREDIENTS:

- 1/4 fueling garlic mashed potato
- 1/2 egg whites
- 1/4 tablespoon baking powder
- 3/4 oz. reduced-fat shredded mozzarella
- 1/8 cup sliced white mushrooms
- 1/16 cup pizza sauce
- 3/4 oz. ground beef
- 1/4 sliced black olives
- You also need a sauté pan, baking sheets, and parchment paper

DIRECTIONS:

1. Start by preheating the oven to 400°F.
2. Mix your baking powder and garlic potato packet.
3. Add egg whites to your mixture and stir well until it blends.
4. Line the baking sheet with parchment paper and pour the mixed batter onto it.
5. Put another parchment paper on top of the batter and spread out the batter to a 1/8-inch circle.
6. Then place another baking sheet on top; this way, the matter is between two baking sheets.
7. Place into an oven and bake for about 8 minutes until the pizza crust is golden brown.
8. For the toppings, place your ground beef in a sauté pan and fry until it's brown and wash your mushrooms very well.
9. After the crust is baked, remove the top layer of parchment paper carefully to prevent the paper from sticking to the pizza crust.
10. Put your toppings on top of the crust and bake for an extra 8 minutes.
11. Once ready, slide the pizza off the parchment paper and into a plate.

NUTRITION :

- Calories: 478
- Protein: 30 g
- Carbohydrates: 22 g
- Fats: 29 g

- **Lean and Green Biscuit Pizza**

Preparation Time: 5 minutes

Cooking Time: 20 minutes

Servings: 1

INGREDIENTS:

- 1/4 sachet buttermilk cheddar and herb biscuit
- 1/4 tablespoon tomato sauce
- 1/4 tablespoon low-fat shredded cheese
- 1/4 table of water
- Parchment paper

DIRECTIONS:

1. You may begin by preheating the oven to about 350°F.
2. Mix the biscuit and water and stir properly.
3. In the parchment paper, pour the mixture and spread it into a thin circle. Allow cooking for 10 minutes.
4. Take it out and add the tomato sauce and shredded cheese.
5. Bake it for a few more minutes.

NUTRITION:

- Calories: 478
- Protein: 30 g
- Carbohydrates: 22 g
- Fats: 29 g

- **Mini Mac in a Bowl**

Preparation Time: 5 minutes

Cooking Time: 15 minutes

Servings: 1

INGREDIENTS:

- 5 oz. lean ground beef
- 2 tablespoons diced white or yellow onion
- 1/8 teaspoon onion powder
- 1/8 teaspoon white vinegar
- 1 oz. dill pickle slices
- 1 teaspoon sesame seed
- 3 cups shredded romaine lettuce
- Cooking spray
- 2 tablespoons reduced-fat shredded cheddar cheese
- 2 tablespoons wish-bone light thousand islands as dressing

DIRECTIONS:

1. Place a lightly greased small skillet on fire to heat.
2. Add your onion to cook for about 2–3 minutes.
3. Next, add the beef and allow it to cook until it is brown.
4. Next, mix your vinegar and onion powder with the dressing.
5. Finally, top the lettuce with the cooked meat and sprinkle cheese on it. Add your pickle slices.
6. Drizzle the mixture with the sauce and sprinkle the sesame seeds also.
7. Your mini mac in a bowl is ready for consumption.

NUTRITION :

- Calories: 150
- Protein: 21 g
- Carbohydrates: 32 g
- Fats: 19 g

- **Lean and Green Smoothie**

Preparation Time: 5 minutes

Cooking Time: 0 minutes

Servings: 1

INGREDIENTS:

- 2 ½ cups of kale leaves
- ¾ cup chilled apple juice
- 1 cup cubed pineapple
- ½ cup frozen green grapes
- ½ cup chopped apple

DIRECTIONS:

1. Place the pineapple, apple juice, apple, frozen seedless grapes, and kale leaves in a blender.

2. Cover and blend until it's smooth.

3. Smoothie is ready and can be garnished with halved grapes if you wish.

NUTRITION:

- Calories: 81
- Protein: 2 g
- Carbohydrates: 19 g
- Fat: 1 g

- **Lean and Green Chicken Pesto Pasta**

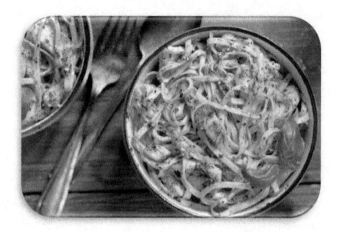

Preparation Time: 5 minutes

Cooking Time: 15 minutes

Servings: 1

INGREDIENTS:

- 3 cups raw kale leaves
- 2 tablespoon olive oil
- 2 cups fresh basil
- ¼ teaspoon salt
- 3 tablespoon lemon juice
- 3 garlic cloves
- 2 cups cooked chicken breast
- 1 cup baby spinach
- 6 oz. uncooked chicken pasta
- 3 oz. diced fresh mozzarella
- Basil leaves or red pepper flakes to garnish

DIRECTIONS:

1. Start by making the pesto, add the kale, lemon juice, basil, garlic cloves, olive oil, and salt to a blender and blend until it is smooth.

2. Add pepper to taste.

3. Cook the pasta and strain off the water. Reserve ¼ cup of the liquid.

4. Get a bowl and mix everything, the cooked pasta, pesto, diced chicken, spinach, mozzarella, and the reserved pasta liquid.

5. Sprinkle the mixture with additional chopped basil or red paper flakes (optional).

6. Now your salad is ready. You may serve it warm or chilled. Also, it can be taken as a salad mix-ins or as a side dish. Leftovers should be stored in the refrigerator inside an airtight container for 3–5 days.

NUTRITION:

- Calories: 244
- Protein: 20.5 g
- Carbohydrates: 22.5 g
- Fats: 10 g

- **Tropical Greens Smoothie**

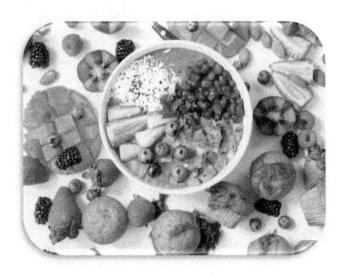

Preparation Time: 5 minutes

Cooking Time: 5 minutes

Servings: 1

INGREDIENTS:

- 1 banana
- 1/2 large navel orange, peeled and segmented
- 1/2 cup frozen mango chunks
- 1 cup frozen spinach
- 1 celery stalk, broken into pieces
- 1 tablespoon cashew butter or almond butter
- 1/2 tablespoon spiraling
- 1/2 tablespoon ground flaxseed
- 1/2 cup unsweetened nondairy milk
- Water, for thinning (optional)

DIRECTIONS:

1. In a high-speed blender or food processor, combine the bananas, orange, mango, spinach, celery, cashew butter, spiraling (if using), flaxseed, and milk.
2. Blend until creamy, adding more milk or water to thin the smoothie if too thick. Serve immediately—it is best served fresh.

NUTRITION:

- Calories: 391
- Fat: 12 g
- Protein: 13 g
- Carbohydrates: 68 g
- Fiber: 13 g

- **Eggless Scramble**

Preparation Time: 10 minutes

Cooking Time: 8 minutes

Servings: 2

INGREDIENTS:

1. 1 tbsp. olive oil
2. 1 garlic clove, minced
3. ¼ lb. medium-firm tofu, drained, pressed, and crumbled
4. 1/3 cup vegetable broth
5. 2¾ cup fresh baby spinach
6. 2 tsp. low-sodium soy sauce
7. 1 tsp. ground turmeric
8. 1 tsp. fresh lemon juice

DIRECTIONS:

1. In a frying pan, heat the olive oil over medium-high heat and sauté the garlic for about 1 minute.
2. Add the tofu and cook for about 2–3 minutes, slowly adding the broth.
3. Add the spinach, soy sauce, and turmeric, and stir fry for about 3–4 minutes or until all the liquid is absorbed.
4. Stir in the lemon juice and remove from the heat.
5. Serve immediately.

NUTRITION:

- Calories per serving: 134
- Carbohydrates: 5.8 g
- Protein: 8.5 g
- Fat: 10.1 g
- Sugar: 1.3 g
- Sodium: 497 mg
- Fiber: 2.7 g

- **Fall Morning Omelet**

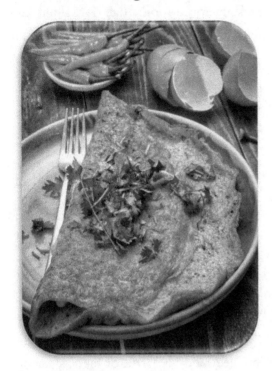

Preparation Time: 10 minutes

Cooking Time: 9 minutes

Servings: 1

INGREDIENTS

- 2 tsp. olive oil, divided
- ½ large green apple, cored and sliced thinly
- ¼ tsp. ground cinnamon
- 1/8 tsp. ground nutmeg
- 2 large eggs
- 1/8 tsp. vanilla extract
- Pinch of salt

DIRECTIONS:

1. In a non-stick frying pan, heat 1 tsp. of oil over medium-low heat.
2. Add apple slices and sprinkle with nutmeg and cinnamon.
3. Cook for about 4–5 minutes, turning once halfway through.
4. Meanwhile, in a bowl, add eggs, vanilla extract, and salt and beat until fluffy.
5. Add the remaining oil to the pan and let it heat completely.
6. Place the egg mixture over apple slices evenly and cook for about 3-4 minutes or until desired doneness.
7. Carefully turn the pan over a serving plate and immediately fold the omelet 8) Serve hot.

NUTRITION:

- Calories per serving: 258
- Carbohydrates: 9 g
- Protein: 12.8 g
- Fat: 19.5 g
- Sugar: 7 g
- Sodium: 295 mg
- Fiber: 1.2 g

- **Delicious Omelet**

Preparation Time: 15 minutes

Cooking Time: 36 minutes

Servings: 2

INGREDIENTS:

- 2 poblano peppers
- Olive oil cooking spray
- 1 small tomato
- ½ tsp. dried oregano
- ½ tsp. chicken bouillon seasoning
- 4 eggs, separated
- 2 tbsp. sour cream
- ½ cup fresh white mushrooms, sliced
- 2/3 cup part-skim mozzarella cheese, shredded and divided

DIRECTIONS:

1. Preheat the oven to the broiler. Line a baking sheet with a piece of foil.
2. Spray the poblano peppers with cooking spray lightly.
3. Arrange the peppers onto the prepared baking sheet in a single layer, and broil for about 5–10 minutes per side or until skin becomes dark ad blistered.
4. Remove from the oven and set aside to cool.
5. After cooking, remove the stems, skin, and seeds from peppers, and then cut each into thin strips.
6. Meanwhile, for the sauce: with a knife, make 2 small slits in a crisscross pattern on the top of the tomato.
7. In a microwave-safe plate, place the tomato and microwave on High for about 2–3 minutes.
8. In a blender, add the tomato, oregano, and chicken bouillon seasoning, and pulse until smooth.
9. Transfer the sauce into a bowl and set aside.
10. In a bowl, add the egg yolks and sour cream and beat until well combined.
11. In a clean glass bowl, add egg whites, and with an electric mixer, beat until soft peaks form.
12. Gently gold the egg yolk mixture into whipped egg whites.
13. Heat a lightly greased skillet over medium-low heat and cook half of the egg mixture cook for about 3–5 minutes or until the bottom is set.
14. Place half of the mushrooms and pepper strips over one half of the omelet and sprinkle with half of the cheese.
15. Cover the skillet and cook for about 2–3 minutes.
16. Uncover the skillet and fold in the omelet.
17. Transfer the omelet onto a plate.
18. Repeat with the remaining egg mixture, mushrooms, pepper strips, and cheese.
19. Top each omelet with sauce and serve.

NUTRITION:

- Calories per serving: 209
- Carbohydrates: 8.4 g
- Protein: 16 g
- Fat: 13.2 g

- Sugar: 4.5 g

- Sodium: 193 mg

- Fiber: 1.6 g

- **Hearty Veggie Omelet**

Preparation Time: 10 minutes

Cooking Time: 25 minutes

Servings: 4

INGREDIENTS:

- 6 large eggs
- ½ cup unsweetened almond milk
- Salt and freshly ground black pepper, to taste
- ½ of onion, chopped
- ¼ cup bell pepper, seeded and chopped
- ¼ cup fresh mushrooms, sliced
- 1 tbsp. chives, minced

DIRECTIONS:

1. Preheat the oven to 350°F. Lightly, grease a pie dish.
2. In a bowl, add eggs, almond milk, salt, and black pepper, and beat until well combined.
3. In a separate bowl, mix together onion, bell pepper, and mushrooms.
4. Place the egg mixture into the prepared pie dish evenly and top with vegetable mixture.
5. Sprinkle with chives evenly.
6. Bake for about 20–25 minutes.
7. Remove the pie dish from the oven and set aside for about 5 minutes.
8. Cut into 4 portions and serve immediately.

NUTRITION:

- Calories per serving: 121
- Carbohydrates: 2.8 g
- Protein: 10 g
- Fat: 8 g
- Sugar: 0.1 g
- Sodium: 167 mg
- Fiber: 0.6 g

- **Earty Veggie Quiche**

Preparation Time: 15 minutes

Cooking Time: 25 minutes

Servings: 4

INGREDIENTS:

- 6 large eggs
- Salt and freshly ground black pepper, to taste
- ½ cup unsweetened almond milk
- ½ of onion, chopped
- ¼ cup fresh mushrooms, cut into slices
- ¼ cup red bell pepper, seeded and diced
- 1 tbsp. fresh chives, minced

DIRECTIONS:

1. Preheat the oven to 350°F. Lightly, grease a pie dish.
2. In a bowl, add the eggs, salt, black pepper, and coconut oil, and beat until well combined.
3. In another bowl, mix together the onion, bell pepper, and mushrooms.
4. Transfer the egg mixture into the prepared pie dish evenly.
5. Top with the vegetable mixture evenly.
6. Sprinkle with chives evenly.
7. Bake for about 20–25 minutes.
8. Remove the pie dish from the oven and set aside for about 5 minutes.
9. Cut into equal-sized wedges and serve.

NUTRITION:

- Calories per serving: 121
- Carbohydrates: 2.9 g
- Protein: 10 g
- Fat: 8 g
- Sugar: 1.6 g
- Sodium: 187 mg
- Fiber: 0.6 g

- **Mushroom Omelet**

Preparation Time: 10 Minutes

Cooking Time: 20 Minutes

Servings: 5

INGREDIENTS:

- 2 spring onions, chopped
- ½ pound white mushrooms
- Salt and black pepper to the taste
- 4 eggs, whisked
- 1 tablespoon olive oil
- ½ teaspoon cumin, ground
- 1 tablespoon cilantro

DIRECTIONS:

1. Heat up a pan with the oil, add the spring onions and the mushrooms, toss and sauté for 5 minutes.

2. Add the eggs and the rest of the ingredients, toss gently, spread into the pan, cover it, and cook over medium heat for 15 minutes.

3. Slice the omelet, divide it between plates, and serve for breakfast.

NUTRITION

- Calories: 109
- Fat: 8.1 g
- Fiber: 0.8 g
- Carbs: 2.9 g
- Protein: 7.5 g

- **Bell Peppers and Avocado Bowls**

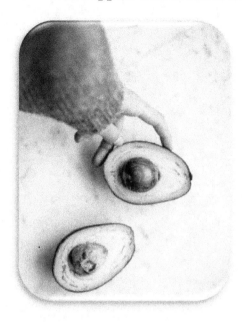

Preparation Time: 10 Minutes

Cooking Time: 15 Minutes

Servings: 5

INGREDIENTS:

- 2 tablespoons olive oil
- 2 shallots, chopped
- 1 red bell pepper, cut into strips
- 1 yellow bell pepper, cut into strips
- 1 green bell pepper, cut into strips
- 1 big avocado, peeled, pitted, and cut into wedges
- 1 teaspoon sweet paprika
- ½ cup vegetable stock
- Salt and black pepper to the taste
- 1 tablespoon chives

DIRECTIONS:

1. Heat up a pan with the oil medium heat, add the shallots and sauté them for 2 minutes.

2. Add the bell peppers, avocado, and the other ingredients except for the chives, toss, bring to a simmer and cook over medium heat for 13 minutes more.

3. Add the chives, toss, divide into bowls, and serve for breakfast.

NUTRITION:

- Calories: 194 g
- Fat: 17.1 g
- Fiber: 4.9 g
- Carbs: 11.5 g
- Protein: 2 g

- **Spinach and Eggs Salad**

Preparation Time: 5 Minutes

Cooking Time: 0 Minutes

Servings: 5

INGREDIENTS:

- 2 cups baby spinach
- 1 cup cherry tomatoes, cubed
- 1 tablespoon chives
- 4 eggs, hard-boiled, peeled, and roughly cubed
- Salt and black pepper to the taste
- 1 tablespoon lime juice
- 1 tablespoon olive oil

DIRECTIONS:

1. In a bowl, combine the spinach with the tomatoes and the other ingredients.
2. Toss and serve for breakfast right away.

NUTRITION:

- Calories: 107
- Fat: 8 g
- Fiber: 0.9 g
- Carbs: 3.6 g
- Protein: 6.4 g

- **Creamy Eggs**

Preparation Time: 10 Minutes

Cooking Time: 15 Minutes

Servings: 5

INGREDIENTS:

- 8 eggs, whisked
- 2 spring onions, chopped
- 1 tablespoon olive oil
- ½ cup heavy cream
- Salt and black pepper to the taste
- ½ cup mozzarella, shredded
- 1 tablespoon chives

DIRECTIONS:

1. Heat up a pan, add the spring onions, toss and sauté them for 3 minutes.

2. Add the eggs mixed with the cream, salt, and pepper and stir into the pan. Sprinkle the mozzarella on top, cook the mix for 12 minutes, divide it between plates, sprinkle the chives on top, and serve.

NUTRITION:

- Calories: 220
- Fat: 18.5 g
- Fiber: 0.2 g
- Carbs: 1.8 g
- Protein: 12.5 g

- **Shrimp and Eggs Mix**

Preparation Time: 5 Minutes

Cooking Time: 11 Minutes

Servings: 5

INGREDIENTS:

- 8 eggs, whisked
- 1 tablespoon olive oil
- ½ pound shrimp, peeled, deveined, and roughly chopped
- ¼ cup green onions, chopped
- 1 teaspoon sweet paprika
- Salt and black pepper to the taste
- 1 tablespoon cilantro

DIRECTIONS:

1. Heat up a pan with the oil, add the spring onions, toss and sauté for 2 minutes.
2. Add the shrimp, stir and cook for 4 minutes more.
3. Add the eggs, paprika, salt, and pepper, toss and cook for 5 minutes more.
4. Divide the mix between plates, sprinkle the cilantro on top, and serve for breakfast.

NUTRITION:

- Calories: 227
- Fat: 13.3 g
- Fiber: 0.4 g
- Carbs: 2.3 g
- Protein: 24.2 g

HEARTY SOUP AND SALADS

- **Taste of Normandy Salad**

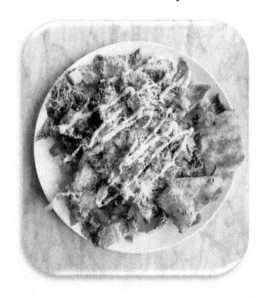

Preparation Time: 25 minutes

Cooking Time: 5 minutes

Servings: 4 to 6

INGREDIENTS:

For the Walnuts:

- 2 tablespoons butter
- ¼ cup sugar or honey
- 1 cup walnut pieces
- ½ teaspoon kosher salt

For the Dressing:

- 3 tablespoons extra-virgin olive oil
- 1½ tablespoons champagne vinegar
- 1½ tablespoons Dijon mustard
- ¼ teaspoon kosher salt

For the Salad:

- 1 head red leaf lettuce, shredded into pieces

- 3 heads endive, ends trimmed and leaves separated
- 2 apples, cored and divided into thin wedges
- 1 (8-ounce) Camembert wheel, cut into thin wedges

DIRECTIONS:

To make the walnuts:

1. Dissolve the butter in a skillet over medium-high heat. Stir in the sugar and cook until it dissolves. Add the walnuts and cook for about 5 minutes, stirring, until toasty. Season with salt and transfer to a plate to cool.

To make the dressing:

2. Whip the oil, vinegar, mustard, and salt in a large bowl until combined.

3. To make the salad

4. Add the lettuce and endive to the bowl with the dressing and toss to coat. Transfer to a serving platter.

5. Decoratively arrange the apple and Camembert wedges over the lettuce and scatter the walnuts on top. Serve immediately.

Meal Prep Tip: Prepare the walnuts in advance—in fact, double the quantities and use them throughout the week to add a healthy crunch to salads, oats, or simply to enjoy as a snack.

NUTRITION:

- Calories: 699
- Total fat: 52 g
- Total carbs: 44 g
- Cholesterol: 60 mg

- Fiber: 17 g
- Protein: 23 g
- Sodium: 1170 mg

- **Shrimp & Arugula Soup**

Preparation Time: 5 Minutes

Cooking Time: 30 Minutes

Servings: 2

INGREDIENTS:

- 10 medium-sized shrimp or 5 large prawns, cleaned, deshelled, and deveined
- 1 small red onion, sliced very thinly
- 1 cup arugula
- 1 cup baby kale
- 2 large celery stalks, sliced very thinly
- 5 sprigs of parsley, chopped
- 11 cloves of garlic, minced
- 5 cups of chicken or fish or vegetable stock
- 1 tbsp. extra virgin olive oil
- Dash of sea salt
- Dash of pepper.

DIRECTIONS:

1. Sauté the vegetables (not the kale or arugula just yet), in a stockpot, on low heat for about 2 minutes so that they are still tender and still crunchy but not cooked quite yet.
2. Add the salt and pepper.
3. Clean and chop the shrimp into bite-sized pieces that would be comfortable eating in a soup.
4. Then, add the shrimp to the pot, and sauté for 10 more minutes on medium-low heat.
5. Make sure the shrimp is cooked thoroughly and is not translucent.
6. When the shrimp seems to be cooked through, add the stock to the pot and cook on medium for about 20 more minutes.
7. Remove from heat and cool before serving.

NUTRITION:

- Calories: 254
- Fat: 2 g
- Carbs: 8 g
- Protein: 33 g
- Sodium: 280 mg

- **Creamy Chicken Soup**

Preparation Time: 10 Minutes

Cooking Time: 30 Minutes

Servings: 2

INGREDIENTS:

- 4 chicken breasts
- 1 carrot, chopped
- 1 cup zucchini, peeled and chopped
- 2 cups cauliflower, broken into florets
- 1 celery rib, chopped
- 1 small onion, chopped
- 5 cups water
- ½ tsp. salt
- Black pepper, to taste

DIRECTIONS:

1. Add in salt, black pepper, and 5 cups of water.
2. Stir and bring to a boil.
3. Blend the soup until completely smooth.
4. Shred or dice the chicken meat, return it back to the pot, stir, and serve.

NUTRITION:

- Calories: 190
- Fat: 2 g
- Carbs: 6 g
- Protein: 26 g
- Sodium: 320mg

- **Broccoli and Chicken Soup**

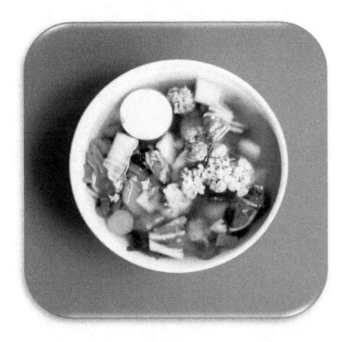

Preparation Time: 5 Minutes

Cooking Time: 30 Minutes

Servings: 2

INGREDIENTS:

- 4 boneless chicken thighs, diced
- 1 small carrot, chopped
- 1 broccoli head, broken into florets
- 1 garlic clove, chopped
- 1 small onion, chopped
- 4 cups water
- 3 tbsp. extra virgin olive oil
- ½ tsp. salt
- Black pepper, to taste

DIRECTIONS:

1. In a deep soup pot, heat olive oil and gently sauté broccoli for 2–3 minutes, stirring occasionally.

2. Add in onion, carrot, chicken, and cook, stirring, for 2–3 minutes. Stir in salt, black pepper, and water.

3. Bring to a boil. Simmer for 30 minutes, then remove from heat and set aside to cool.

4. In a blender or food processor, blend soup until completely smooth.

NUTRITION:

- Calories: 185 g
- Fat: 2 g
- Carbs: 4 g
- Protein: 22 g
- Sodium: 564 mg

- **Warm Chicken and Avocado Soup**

Preparation Time: 5 Minutes

Cooking Time: 30 Minutes

Servings: 2

INGREDIENTS:

- 2 ripe avocados, peeled and chopped
- 1 cooked chicken breast, shredded
- 1 garlic clove, chopped
- 3 cups chicken broth
- Salt and black pepper, to taste
- Fresh coriander leaves, finely cut, to serve
- ½ cup sour cream, to serve

DIRECTIONS:

1. Combine avocados, garlic, and chicken broth in a blender.
2. Process until smooth and transfer to a saucepan. Add in chicken and cook, stirring, over medium heat until the mixture is hot. Serve topped with sour cream and finely cut coriander leaves

NUTRITION:

- Calories: 480
- Fat: 2 g
- Carbs: 8 g
- Protein: 42 g
- Sodium: 643 g

- **Loaded Caesar Salad with Crunchy Chickpeas**

Preparation Time: 5 minutes

Cooking Time: 20 minutes

Servings: 6

INGREDIENT:

For the Chickpeas:

- 2 (15-ounce) cans chickpeas, drained and rinsed
- 2 tablespoons extra-virgin olive oil
- 1 teaspoon kosher salt
- 1 teaspoon garlic powder
- 1 teaspoon onion powder
- 1 teaspoon dried oregano

For the Dressing:

- ½ cup mayonnaise
- 2 tablespoons grated Parmesan cheese
- 2 tablespoons freshly squeezed lemon juice
- 1 clove garlic, peeled and smashed
- 1 teaspoon Dijon mustard
- ½ tablespoon Worcestershire sauce
- ½ tablespoon anchovy paste

For the Salad:

- 3 heads romaine lettuce, cut into bite-size pieces

DIRECTIONS:

To make the chickpeas:

1. Preheat the oven to 450°F. Line a baking sheet with parchment paper.

2. Add the chickpeas, oil, salt, garlic powder, onion powder, and oregano in a small container. Scatter the coated chickpeas on the prepared baking sheet.

3. Roast for about 20 minutes, tossing occasionally, until the chickpeas are golden and have a bit of crunch.

To make the dressing:

4. In a small bowl, whisk the mayonnaise, Parmesan, lemon juice, garlic, mustard, Worcestershire sauce, and anchovy paste until combined.

To make the salad:

5. Combine the lettuce and dressing in a large container. Toss to coat. Top with the roasted chickpeas and serve.

Cooking Tip: Don't wash out that bowl you used for the chickpeas—the remaining oil adds a great punch of flavor to blanched green beans or another simply cooked vegetable.

NUTRITION:

- Calories: 367
- Total fat: 22 g
- Total carbs: 35 g
- Cholesterol: 9 mg
- Fiber: 13 g
- Protein: 12 g
- Sodium: 407 mg

- **Coleslaw Worth a Second Helping**

Preparation Time: 20 minutes

Cooking Time: 10 minutes

Servings: 6

INGREDIENTS:

- 5 cups shredded cabbage
- 2 carrots, shredded
- ½ cup mayonnaise
- ½ cup sour cream
- 3 tablespoons apple cider vinegar
- 1 teaspoon kosher salt
- ½ teaspoon celery seed

DIRECTIONS:

1. Add together the cabbage, carrots, and parsley in a large bowl.

2. Whisk together the mayonnaise, sour cream, vinegar, salt, and celery in a small bowl until smooth. Pour sauce over veggies and pour until covered. Transfer to a serving bowl and bake until ready to serve.

NUTRITION:

- Calories: 192
- Total fat: 18 g
- Total carbs: 7 g
- Cholesterol: 18 mg
- Fiber: 3 g
- Protein: 2 g
- Sodium: 543 mg

- **Romaine Lettuce and Radicchios Mix**

Preparation Time: 6 minutes

Cooking Time: 0 minutes

Servings: 4

INGREDIENTS:

- 2 tablespoons olive oil
- A pinch of salt and black pepper
- 2 spring onions, chopped
- 3 tablespoons Dijon mustard
- Juice of 1 lime
- ½ cup basil, chopped
- 4 cups romaine lettuce heads, chopped
- 3 radicchios, sliced

DIRECTIONS:

1. In a salad bowl, blend the lettuce with the spring onions and the other ingredients, toss and serve.

NUTRITION:

- Calories: 87
- Fats: 2 g
- Fiber: 1 g
- Carbs: 1 g
- Protein: 2 g

- **Greek Salad**

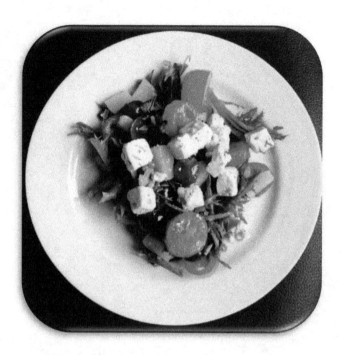

Preparation Time: 15 Minutes.

Cooking Time: 15 Minutes.

Servings: 5.

INGREDIENTS:

For Dressing:

- ½ teaspoon black pepper.
- ¼ teaspoon salt.
- ½ teaspoon oregano.
- 1 tablespoon garlic powder.
- 2 tablespoons Balsamic.
- 1/3 cup olive oil.

For Salad:

- ½ cup sliced black olives.
- ½ cup chopped parsley, fresh.
- 1 small red onion, thin-sliced.
- 1 cup cherry tomatoes, sliced.

- 1 bell pepper, yellow, chunked.
- 1 cucumber, peeled, quarter and slice.
- 4 cups chopped romaine lettuce.
- ½ teaspoon salt.
- 2 tablespoons olive oil.

DIRECTIONS

1. In a small container, join all of the ingredients for the dressing and let this set in the freezer while you make the salad.

2. To assemble the salad, mix together all the ingredients in a large-sized bowl and toss the veggies gently but thoroughly to mix.

3. Serve the salad with the dressing in amounts as desired.

NUTRITION:

- Calories: 234.
- Fat: 16.1 g.
- Protein: 5 g.
- Carbs: 48 g.

- **Asparagus and Smoked Salmon Salad**

Preparation Time: 15 minutes.

Cooking Time: 10 minutes.

Servings: 8.

INGREDIENTS:

- 1 lb. fresh asparagus, shaped and cut into 1-inch pieces.

- 1/2 cup pecans, smashed into pieces.

- 2 heads red leaf lettuce, washed and split.

- 1/2 cup frozen green peas, thawed.

- 1/4 lb. smoked salmon, cut into 1-inch chunks.

- 1/4 cup olive oil.

- 2 tablespoons. lemon juice.

- 1 teaspoon Dijon mustard.

- 1/2 teaspoon salt.

- 1/4 teaspoon pepper.

DIRECTIONS:

1. Boil a pot of water. Stir in asparagus and cook for 5 minutes until tender. Let it drain; set aside.

2. In a skillet, cook the pecans over medium heat for 5 minutes, constantly stirring until lightly toasted.

3. Combine the asparagus, toasted pecans, salmon, peas, and red leaf lettuce and toss in a large bowl.

4. In another bowl, combine lemon juice, pepper, Dijon mustard, salt, and olive oil. You can coat the salad with the dressing or serve it on its side.

NUTRITION:

- Calories: 159.

- Total Carbohydrate: 7 g.

- Cholesterol: 3 mg.

- Total Fat: 12.9 g.

- Protein: 6 g.

- Sodium: 304 mg.

- **Shrimp Cobb Salad**

Preparation Time: 25 minutes.

Cooking Time: 10 minutes.

Servings: 2.

INGREDIENTS

- 4 slices center-cut bacon.

- 1 lb. large shrimp, peeled and deveined.

- 1/2 teaspoon ground paprika.

- 1/4 teaspoon ground black pepper.

- 1/4 teaspoon salt, divided.

- 2 1/2 tablespoons Fresh lemon juice.

- 1 1/2 tablespoons Extra-virgin olive oil.

- 1/2 teaspoon whole-grain Dijon mustard.

- 1 (10 oz.) package romaine lettuce hearts, chopped.

- 2 cups cherry tomatoes, quartered.

- 1 ripe avocado, cut into wedges.

- 1 cup shredded carrots.

DIRECTIONS:

1. Cook the bacon for 4 minutes on each side in a large skillet over medium heat till crispy.

2. Take away from the skillet and place on paper towels; let cool for 5 minutes. Break the bacon into bits. Throw out most of the bacon fat, leaving behind only 1 tablespoon in the skillet. Bring the skillet back to medium-high heat. Add black pepper and paprika to the shrimp for seasoning. Cook the shrimp around 2 minutes on each side until it is opaque. Sprinkle with 1/8 teaspoon of salt for seasoning.

3. Combine the remaining 1/8 teaspoon of salt, mustard, olive oil, and lemon juice together in a small bowl. Stir in the romaine hearts.

4. On each serving plate, place 1 and 1/2 cups of romaine lettuce. Add on top the same amounts of avocado, carrots, tomatoes, shrimp, and bacon.

NUTRITION:

- Calories: 528.

- Total Carbohydrate: 22.7 g.

- Cholesterol: 365 mg.

- Total Fat: 28.7 g.

- Protein: 48.9 g.

- Sodium: 1166 mg.

- **Avocado, Citrus, and Shrimp Salad**

Preparation Time: 15 Minutes.

Cooking Time: 0 Minutes.

Servings: 2.

INGREDIENTS:

- 1 head green leaf lettuce.

- 1 avocado.

- ½ pound wild-caught shrimp.

- 2 tablespoons olive oil.

- Juice of 1 lemon.

DIRECTIONS:

1. Place the lettuce in a bowl and top with mashed avocado meat.

2. Clean the shrimps by deveining and removing the head.

3. Heat oil in a skillet over medium-low heat and heat the oil. Cook the shrimps for 2 minutes on each side.

4. Place the shrimps on top of mashed avocado and drizzle with lemon juice.

NUTRITION:

- Calories 359.

- Fat 5 g.

- Carbs 16 g.

- Protein 6 g.

- Sodium 585 g.

- **Healthy Salmon Salad**

Preparation Time: 10 Minutes.

Cooking Time: 0 Minutes.

Servings: 2.

INGREDIENTS:

- 2 salmon fillets
- 2 tbsp olive oil
- ¼ cup onion, chopped
- 1 cucumber, peeled and sliced
- 1 avocado, diced
- 2 tomatoes, chopped
- 4 cups baby spinach
- Pepper
- Salt

DIRECTIONS:

1. Heat oil in a pan over medium-high heat.
2. Season salmon fillets with pepper and salt. Place fish fillets in a pan and cook for 4–5 minutes.
3. Turn fish fillets and cook for 2–3 minutes more.
4. Divide remaining ingredients evenly between two bowls, then top with cooked fish fillet.

NUTRITION:

- Calories 320.
- Fat 8 g.
- Carbs 21 g.
- Protein 8 g.
- Sodium 650 g.

- **Strawberry, Apple & Arugula Salad**

Preparation Time: 10 Minutes.

Cooking Time: 0 Minutes.

Servings: 2.

INGREDIENTS

- 4 cups fresh baby arugula.

- 2 apples, cored and sliced.

- 1 cup fresh strawberries, hulled and sliced.

- ¼ cup walnuts, chopped.

- 4 tablespoons olive oil.

- Salt and ground black pepper, as required.

DIRECTIONS:

1. For the salad, place all the ingredients in a large bowl and mix well.

2. For the dressing, place all the ingredients in a bowl and beat until well combined.

3. Pour the dressing over the salad and toss it all to coat thoroughly.

4. Serve immediately.

NUTRITION:

- Calories: 350.

- Fat: 2 g.

- Carbs: 8 g.

- Protein: 6 g.

- Sodium: 397 g.

- **Raspberry & Kale Salad**

Preparation Time: 15 Minutes.

Cooking Time: 0 Minutes.

Servings: 2.

INGREDIENTS

For Salad:

- 3 cups fresh baby kale.
- ½ cup fresh raspberries.
- ¼ cup walnuts, chopped.

For Dressing:

- 1 tablespoon extra-virgin olive oil.
- 1 tablespoon apple cider vinegar.
- ½ teaspoon pure maple syrup.
- Salt and ground black pepper, as required.

DIRECTIONS:

For salad:

1. In a salad bowl, place all ingredients and mix.

For dressing:

2. Place all ingredients in another bowl and beat until well combined.
3. Place dressing on top of the salad and toss to coat thoroughly.
4. Serve immediately.

NUTRITION:

- Calories: 486 g.
- Fat: 1 g.
- Carbs: 2 g.
- Protein: 16 g.
- Sodium: 690 g.

- **Cucumber & Onion Salad**

Preparation Time: 10 Minutes.

Cooking Time: 0 Minutes.

Servings: 2.

INGREDIENTS

- 3 large cucumbers, sliced thinly.
- ½ cup red onion, sliced.
- 2 tablespoons olive oil.
- 1 tablespoon fresh apple cider vinegar.
- Sea salt, to taste.
- ¼ cup fresh parsley, chopped.

DIRECTIONS:

1. In a salad bowl, place all the ingredients and toss to coat thoroughly.
2. Serve immediately.

NUTRITION:

- Calories: 254.
- Fat: 1 g.
- Carbs: 2 g.
- Protein: 14 g.
- Sodium: 321 g.

- **Shrimp Salad**

Preparation Time: 15 Minutes.

Cooking Time: 5 Minutes.

Servings: 2.

INGREDIENTS:

For Shrimp:

- 1 tablespoon olive oil.
- 1 garlic clove, crushed.
- 2 tablespoons fresh rosemary, chopped.
- 1-pound raw shrimp, peeled and deveined.
- ¼ teaspoon red pepper flakes, crushed.
- Salt and ground black pepper, as required.

For Salad:

- 8 cups fresh arugula.
- 3 tablespoons olive oil.
- 2 tablespoons fresh lime juice.
- Salt and ground black pepper, as required.

DIRECTIONS:

1. In a large wok, heat oil over medium heat and sauté 1 garlic clove for about 1 minute.
2. Add the shrimp with red pepper flakes, salt, and black pepper and cook for about 4-5 minutes.
3. Remove the wok of shrimp from heat and set aside to cool.
4. In a large bowl, add the shrimp, arugula, oil, lime juice, salt, and black pepper, and gently toss to coat.
5. Serve immediately.

NUTRITION:

- Calories: 190.
- Fat: 2 g.
- Carbs: 8 g.
- Protein: 8 g.

- **Chicken Cobb Salad**

Preparation Time: 10 Minutes.

Cooking Time: 0 Minutes.

Servings: 2.

INGREDIENTS

- ½ lb. cooked chicken breast, cubed or sliced.
- 2 hard-boiled eggs, sliced.
- 1 cup cherry tomatoes, halved.
- 2 slices cooked turkey bacon, chopped.
- ¼ cup nonfat. Plain Greek yogurt.
- 1/4 avocado, mashed.
- 1 tsp dry rant mix.
- Water to thin.
- 1 sachet Puffed Ranch Snacks.

DIRECTIONS:

1. Divide remaining salad toppings amongst both salad bowls.

To prepare the dressing:

2. Combine yogurt, avocado, ranch mix, and water in a small bowl, and mix until smooth.

3. Top salads with dressing and Puffed Ranch Snacks, and serve immediately.

NUTRITION:

- Calories: 190.
- Fat: 2 g.
- Carbs: 8 g.
- Protein: 8 g.
- Sodium: 231 g.

- **Curried Chicken Salad Wraps**

Preparation Time: 5 Minutes.

Cooking Time: 0 Minutes.

Servings: 2.

INGREDIENTS:

- 1 (10 oz.) chicken breast, packed in water.
- ½ cup low fat plain Greek yogurt.
- 1/2 cup diced celery.
- 2 tsp. curry powder.
- 2 tbsp. fresh parsley chopped.
- 1/4 tsp. salt.
- ¼ tsp. ground pepper.
- 8 large green leaf or romaine lettuce leaves.
- 2/3 oz. chopped peanuts.

DIRECTIONS:

1. Mix the chicken, yogurt, celery, herbs, and spices together in a medium bowl.

NUTRITION:

- Calories: 190.
- Fat: 2 g.
- Carbs: 8 g.
- Protein: 8 g.
- Sodium: 231 g.

- **Asparagus Avocado Soup**

Preparation Time: 5 Minutes.

Cooking Time: 30 Minutes.

Servings: 2.

INGREDIENTS

- 1 avocado, peeled, pitted, and cubed.

- 12 ounces asparagus.

- ½ teaspoon ground black pepper.

- 1 teaspoon garlic powder.

- 1 teaspoon sea salt.

- 2 tablespoons olive oil, divided.

- 1/2 of a lemon, juiced.

- 2 cups vegetable stock.

DIRECTIONS:

1. Set the fryer at 425°F and preheat for 5 minutes.

2. Meanwhile, place asparagus in a shallow dish, drizzle with 1 tablespoon oil, sprinkle with garlic powder, salt, and black pepper, and toss until well mixed.

3. Open the fryer, add asparagus to it, close with its lid and cook for 10 minutes until nicely golden and roasted, shaking halfway through the frying.

4. When the air fryer beeps, open its lid and transfer asparagus to a food processor.

5. Add remaining ingredients into a food processor and pulse until well combined and smooth.

6. Tip the soup in a saucepan, pour in water if the soup is too thick, and heat it over medium-low heat for 5 minutes until thoroughly heated.

7. Ladle soup into bowls and serve.

NUTRITION:

- Calories: 208.

- Carbs: 2 g.

- Fat: 11 g.

- Protein: 4 g.

- Fiber: 5 g.

- **Arugula and Broccoli Soup**

Preparation Time: 10 Minutes.

Cooking Time: 25 Minutes.

Servings: 5.

INGREDIENTS:

- 1 small yellow onion, chopped.
- 1 tablespoon olive oil.
- 1 garlic clove, minced.
- 1 broccoli head, florets separated.
- Salt and black pepper to the taste.
- 2 and ½ cups veggie stock.
- 1 teaspoon cumin, ground.
- Juice from ½ lemon.
- 1 cup arugula leaves.

DIRECTIONS:

1. Heat up a pot with the oil over medium-high heat, add onions, stir and cook for 4 minutes.
2. Add garlic, stir and cook for 1 minute.
3. Add broccoli, cumin, salt, and pepper. Stir and cook for 4 minutes.
4. Add stock, stir and cook for 8 minutes.
5. Blend soup using an immersion blender, add half of the arugula and blend again.
6. Add the rest of the arugula, stir, and heat up the soup again.
7. Add lemon juice, stir, ladle into soup bowls and serve.
8. Enjoy!

NUTRITION:

- Calories: 150.
- Fat: 3 g.
- Fiber: 1 g.
- Carbs: 3 g.
- Protein: 7 g.

- **Delicious Zucchini Cream**

Preparation Time: 10 Minutes.

Cooking Time: 25 Minutes.

Servings: 8.

INGREDIENTS:

- 6 zucchinis, cut in halves and then sliced.
- Salt and black pepper to the taste.
- 1 tablespoon ghee.
- 28 ounces veggie stock.
- 1 teaspoon oregano, dried.
- ½ cup yellow onion, chopped.
- 3 garlic cloves, minced.
- 2 ounces parmesan, grated.
- ¾ cup heavy cream.

DIRECTIONS:

1. Heat up a pot with the ghee over medium-high heat, add onion, stir and cook for 4 minutes.
2. Add garlic, stir and cook for 2 minutes more.
3. Add zucchinis, stir and cook for 3 minutes.
4. Add stock, stir, bring to a boil and simmer over medium heat for 15 minutes.
5. Add oregano, salt, and pepper, stir, take off heat, and blend using an immersion blender.
6. Heat up soup again, add heavy cream, stir and bring to a simmer.
7. Add parmesan, stir, take off heat, ladle into bowls, and serve right away.
8. Enjoy!

NUTRITION:

- Calories 160.
- Fat 4 g.
- Fiber 2 g.
- Carbs 4 g.
- Protein: 8 g.

- **Zucchini and Avocado Soup**

Preparation Time: 10 Minutes.

Cooking Time: 15 Minutes.

Servings: 5.

INGREDIENTS:

- 1 big avocado, pitted, peeled, and chopped
- 4 scallions, chopped
- 1 teaspoon ginger, grated
- 2 tablespoons avocado oil
- Salt and black pepper to the taste
- 2 zucchinis, chopped.
- 29 ounces veggie stock
- 1 garlic clove, minced
- 1 cup water.
- 1 tablespoon lemon juice
- 1 red bell pepper, chopped.

DIRECTIONS:

1. Heat up a pot with the oil over medium heat, add onions, stir and cook for 3 minutes.

2. Add garlic and ginger, stir and cook for 1 minute.

3. Add zucchini, salt, pepper, water, and stock, stir, bring to a boil, cover pot and cook for 10 minutes.

4. Take off heat, leave soup aside for a couple of minutes, add avocado, stir, and blend everything using an immersion blender and heat up again.

5. Add more salt and pepper, bell pepper, and lemon juice, stir, heat up soup again, ladle into soup bowls and serve.

6. Enjoy!

NUTRITION:

- Calories: 154 g.
- Fat: 12 g.
- Fiber: 3 g.
- Carbs: 5 g.
- Protein: 4 g.

- **Swiss Chard Pie**

Preparation Time: 10 Minutes.

Cooking Time: 45 Minutes.

Servings: 12.

INGREDIENTS:

- 8 cups Swiss chard, chopped.
- ½ cup onion, chopped.
- 1 tablespoon olive oil.
- 1 garlic clove, minced.
- Salt and black pepper to the taste.
- 3 eggs.
- 2 cups ricotta cheese.
- 1 cup mozzarella, shredded.
- A pinch of nutmeg.
- ¼ cup parmesan, grated.
- 1 pound sausage, chopped.

DIRECTIONS:

1. Heat up a pan with the oil over medium heat, add onions and garlic, stir and cook for 3 minutes.
2. Add Swiss chard, stir and cook for 5 minutes more.
3. Add salt, pepper, and nutmeg, stir, take off the heat and leave aside for a few minutes.
4. In a bowl, whisk eggs with mozzarella, parmesan, and ricotta and stir well.
5. Add Swiss chard mix and stir well.
6. Spread sausage meat on the bottom of a pie pan and press well.
7. Add Swiss chard and eggs mix, spread well, introduce in the oven at 350°F and bake for 35 minutes.
8. Leave pie aside to cool down, slice, and serve it.
9. Enjoy!

NUTRITION:

- Calories: 332.
- Fat: 23 g.
- Fiber: 3 g.
- Carbs: 4 g.
- Protein: 23 g.

- **Swiss Chard Salad**

- Protein: 8 g.

Preparation Time: 10 Minutes.

Cooking Time: 20 Minutes.

Servings: 5.

INGREDIENTS:

- 1 bunch Swiss chard, cut in strips.

- 2 tablespoons avocado oil.

- 1 small yellow onion, chopped.

- A pinch of red pepper flakes.

- ¼ cup pine nuts, toasted.

- ¼ cup raisins.

- 1 tablespoon balsamic vinegar.

- Salt and black pepper to the taste.

DIRECTIONS:

1. Heat up a pan with the oil over medium heat, add chard and onions, stir and cook for 5 minutes.

2. Add salt, pepper, and pepper flakes, stir and cook for 3 minutes more.

3. Put raisins in a bowl, add water to cover them, heat them up in your microwave for 1 minute, leave aside for 5 minutes, and drain them well.

4. Add raisins and pine nuts to the pan, also add vinegar, stir, cook for 3 minutes more, divide into plates and serve.

5. Enjoy!

NUTRITION:

- Calories: 120.

- Fat: 2 g.

- Fiber: 1 g.

- Carbs: 4 g.

SIDE DISHES AND SNACKS

- **Parmesan Sweet Potato Casserole**

Preparation Time: 15 Minutes.

Cooking Time: 35 Minutes.

Servings: 2.

INGREDIENTS:

- 2 sweet potatoes, peeled.
- ½ yellow onion, sliced.
- ½ cup cream.
- ¼ cup spinach.
- 2 oz. Parmesan cheese, shredded.
- ½ teaspoon salt.
- 1 tomato.
- 1 teaspoon olive oil.

DIRECTIONS:

1. Chop the sweet potatoes, the tomato, and the spinach.
2. Spray the air fryer tray with the olive oil.
3. Then place on the layer of the chopped sweet potato.
4. Add the layer of the sliced onion.
5. After this, sprinkle the sliced onion with the chopped spinach and tomatoes.
6. Sprinkle the casserole with the salt and the shredded cheese, then pour the cream.
7. Preheat the air fryer to 390°F.
8. Cover the air fryer tray with the foil.
9. Cook the casserole for 35 minutes.
10. When the casserole is cooked, serve it.
11. Enjoy!

NUTRITION:

- Calories: 93.
- Fat: 1.8 g.
- Fiber: 3.4 g.
- Carbs: 20.3 g.
- Protein: 1.8 g.

- **Spicy Zucchini Slices**

Preparation Time: 10 Minutes.

Cooking Time: 6 Minutes.

Servings: 2.

INGREDIENTS:

- 1 teaspoon cornstarch.
- 1 zucchini.
- ½ teaspoon chili flakes.
- 1 tablespoon flour.
- 1 egg.
- ¼ teaspoon salt.

DIRECTIONS:

1. Slice the zucchini and sprinkle with the chili flakes and salt.
2. Crack the egg into the bowl and whisk it.
3. Dip the zucchini slices into the whisked egg.
4. Combine cornstarch with the flour. Stir it.
5. Coat the zucchini slices with the cornstarch mixture.
6. Preheat the air fryer to 400°F.
7. Place the zucchini slices in the air fryer tray, and cook the zucchini slices for four minutes.
8. After this, flip the slices to the other side and cook for 2 minutes more.
9. Serve the zucchini slices hot.
10. Enjoy!

NUTRITION:

- Calories: 67.
- Fat: 2.4 g.
- Fiber: 1.2 g.
- Carbs: 7.7 g.
- Protein: 4.4 g.

- **Cheddar Potato Gratin**

Preparation Time: 15 Minutes.

Cooking Time: 20 Minutes.

Servings: 2.

INGREDIENTS:

- 2 potatoes.
- 1/3 cup half and half.
- 1 tablespoon oatmeal flour.
- ¼ teaspoon ground black pepper.
- 1 egg.
- 2 oz. Cheddar cheese.

DIRECTIONS:

1. Wash the potatoes and slice them into thin pieces.
2. Preheat the air fryer to 365°F.
3. Put the potato slices in the air fryer and cook them for 10 minutes.
4. Meanwhile, combine the half and half, oatmeal flour, and ground black pepper.
5. Crack the egg into the liquid and whisk it carefully, then shred the cheddar cheese.
6. When the potato is cooked, take 2 ramekins and place the potatoes on them.
7. Pour the half and half mixture.
8. Sprinkle the gratin with shredded Cheddar cheese.
9. Cook the gratin for 10 minutes at 360°F.
10. Serve the meal immediately.
11. Enjoy!

NUTRITION:

- Calories: 353.
- Fat: 16.6 g.
- Fiber: 5.4 g.
- Carbs: 37.2 g.
- Protein: 15 g.

- **Salty Lemon Artichokes**

Preparation Time: 15 Minutes.

Cooking Time: 45 Minutes.

Servings: 2.

INGREDIENTS:

- 1 lemon.
- 2 artichokes.
- 1 teaspoon kosher salt.
- 1 garlic head.
- 2 teaspoons olive oil.

DIRECTIONS:

1. Cut off the edges of the artichokes.
2. Cut the lemon into halves.
3. Peel the garlic head and chop the garlic cloves roughly.
4. Then place the chopped garlic in the artichokes.
5. Sprinkle the artichokes with olive oil and kosher salt.
6. Then squeeze the lemon juice into the artichokes.
7. Wrap the artichokes in the foil.
8. Preheat the air fryer to 330°F.
9. Place the wrapped artichokes in the air fryer and cook for 45 minutes.
10. When the artichokes are cooked, discard the foil and serve.
11. Enjoy!

NUTRITION:

- Calories: 133.
- Fat: 5 g.
- Fiber: 9.7 g.
- Carbs: 21.7 g.
- Protein: 6 g.

- **Asparagus & Parmesan**

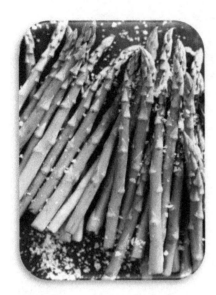

Preparation Time: 10 Minutes.

Cooking Time: 6 Minutes.

Servings: 2.

INGREDIENTS:

- 1 teaspoon sesame oil.

- 11 oz. Asparagus.

- 1 teaspoon chicken stock.

- ½ teaspoon ground white pepper.

- 3 oz. Parmesan.

DIRECTIONS:

1. Wash the asparagus and chop them roughly.

2. Sprinkle the chopped asparagus with the chicken stock and ground white pepper.

3. Then sprinkle the vegetables with the sesame oil and shake them.

4. Place the asparagus in the air fryer's basket.

5. Cook the vegetables for 4 minutes at 400°F.

6. Meanwhile, shred Parmesan cheese.

7. When the time is over, shake the asparagus gently and sprinkle with the shredded cheese.

8. Cook the asparagus for 2 minutes more at 400°F.

9. After this, transfer the cooked asparagus to the serving plates.

10. Serve and taste it!

NUTRITION:

- Calories: 189.

- Fat: 11.6 g.

- Fiber: 3.4 g.

- Carbs: 7.9 g.

- Protein: 17.2 g.

- **Carrot Lentil Burgers**

Preparation Time: 10 Minutes.

Cooking Time: 15 Minutes.

Servings: 2.

INGREDIENTS:

- 6 oz. lentils, cooked.
- 1 egg.
- 2 oz. carrot, grated.
- 1 teaspoon semolina.
- ½ teaspoon salt.
- 1 teaspoon turmeric.
- 1 tablespoon butter.

DIRECTIONS:

1. Crack the egg into the bowl and whisk it.
2. Add the cooked lentils and mash the mixture with the help of the fork.
3. Then sprinkle the mixture with the grated carrot, semolina, salt, and turmeric.
4. Mix it up and make the medium burgers.
5. Put the butter into the lentil burgers. It will make them juicy.
6. Preheat the air fryer to 360°F.
7. Put the lentil burgers in the air fryer and cook for 12 minutes.
8. Flip the burgers into another side after 6 minutes of cooking.
9. Then chill the cooked lentil burgers and serve them.
10. Enjoy!

NUTRITION:

- Calories: 404.
- Fat: 9 g.
- Fiber: 26.9 g.
- Carbs: 56 g.
- Protein: 25.3 g.

- **Corn on Cobs**

Preparation Time: 10 Minutes.

Cooking Time: 10 Minutes.

Servings: 2.

INGREDIENTS:

- 2 fresh corn on cobs.

- 2 teaspoon butter.

- 1 teaspoon salt.

- 1 teaspoon paprika.

- ¼ teaspoon olive oil.

DIRECTIONS:

1. Preheat the air fryer to 400°F.

2. Rub the corn on cobs with the salt and paprika.

3. Then sprinkle the corn on cobs with olive oil.

4. Place the corn on cobs in the air fryer's basket.

5. Cook the corn on cobs for 10 minutes.

6. When the time is over, transfer the corn on cobs to the serving plates and rub with the butter gently.

7. Serve the meal immediately.

8. Enjoy!

NUTRITION:

- Calories: 122.

- Fat: 5.5 g.

- Fiber: 2.4 g.

- Carbs: 17.6 g.

- Protein: 3.2 g.

- **Sugary Carrot Strips**

Preparation Time: 10 Minutes.

Cooking Time: 10 Minutes.

Servings: 2.

INGREDIENTS:

- 2 carrots.

- 1 teaspoon brown sugar.

- 1 teaspoon olive oil.

- 1 tablespoon soy sauce.

- 1 teaspoon honey.

- ½ teaspoon ground black pepper.

DIRECTIONS:

1. Peel the carrot and cut it into strips.

2. Then put the carrot strips in the bowl.

3. Sprinkle the carrot strips with the olive oil, soy sauce, honey, and ground black pepper.

4. Shake the mixture gently.

5. Preheat the air fryer to 360°F.

6. Cook the carrot for 10 minutes.

7. After this, shake the carrot strips well.

8. Enjoy!

NUTRITION:

- Calories: 67.

- Fat: 2.4 g.

- Fiber: 1.7 g.

- Carbs: 11.3 g.

- Protein: 1.1 g.

- **Onion Green Beans**

Preparation Time: 10 Minutes.

Cooking Time: 15 Minutes.

Servings: 2.

INGREDIENTS:

- 11 oz. green beans.

- 1 tablespoon onion powder.

- 1 tablespoon olive oil.

- ½ teaspoon salt.

- ¼ teaspoon chili flakes.

DIRECTIONS:

1. Wash the green beans carefully and place them in the bowl.

2. Sprinkle the green beans with the onion powder, salt, chili flakes, and olive oil.

3. Shake the green beans carefully.

4. Preheat the air fryer to 400°F.

5. Put the green beans in the air fryer and cook for 8 minutes.

6. After this, shake the green beans and cook them for 4 minutes more at 400°F.

7. When the time is over, shake the green beans.

8. Serve the side dish and enjoy!

NUTRITION:

- Calories: 1205.

- Fat: 7.2 g.

- Fiber: 5.5 g.

- Carbs: 13.9 g.

- Protein: 3.2 g.

- **Mozzarella Radish Salad**

Preparation Time: 10 Minutes.

Cooking Time: 20 Minutes.

Servings: 2.

INGREDIENTS:

- 8 oz. Radish.

- 4 oz. Mozzarella.

- 1 teaspoon balsamic vinegar.

- ½ teaspoon salt.

- 1 tablespoon olive oil.

- 1 teaspoon dried oregano.

DIRECTIONS:

1. Wash the radish carefully and cut it into halves.

2. Preheat the air fryer to 360°F.

3. Put the radish halves in the air fryer basket.

4. Sprinkle the radish with salt and olive oil.

5. Cook the radish for 20 minutes.

6. Shake the radish after 10 minutes of cooking.

7. When the time is over, transfer the radish to the serving plate.

8. Chop Mozzarella roughly.

9. Sprinkle the radish with Mozzarella, balsamic vinegar, and dried oregano.

10. Stir it gently using two forks.

11. Serve it immediately.

NUTRITION:

- Calories: 241.

- Fat: 17.2 g.

- Fiber: 2.1 g.

- Carbs: 6.4 g.

- Protein: 16.9 g.

- **Cremini Mushroom Satay**

Preparation Time: 10 Minutes.

Cooking Time: 6 Minutes.

Servings: 2.

INGREDIENTS:

- 7 oz. cremini mushrooms.
- 2 tablespoon coconut milk.
- 1 tablespoon butter.
- 1 teaspoon chili flakes.
- ½ teaspoon balsamic vinegar.
- ½ teaspoon curry powder.
- ½ teaspoon white pepper.

DIRECTIONS:

1. Wash the mushrooms carefully.
2. Then sprinkle the mushrooms with chili flakes, curry powder, and white pepper.
3. Preheat the air fryer to 400°F.
4. Toss the butter in the air fryer basket and melt it.
5. Put the mushrooms in the air fryer and cook for 2 minutes.
6. Shake the mushrooms well and sprinkle with the coconut milk and balsamic vinegar.
7. Cook the mushrooms for 4 minutes more at 400°F.
8. Then skewer the mushrooms on the wooden sticks and serve.
9. Enjoy!

NUTRITION:

- Calories: 116.
- Fat: 9.5 g.
- Fiber: 1.3 g.
- Carbs: 5.6 g.
- Protein: 3 g.

- **Eggplant Ratatouille**

Preparation Time: 15 Minutes.

Cooking Time: 15 Minutes.

Servings: 2.

INGREDIENTS:

- 1 eggplant.
- 1 sweet yellow pepper.
- 3 cherry tomatoes.
- 1/3 white onion, chopped.
- ½ teaspoon garlic clove, sliced.
- 1 teaspoon olive oil.
- ½ teaspoon ground black pepper.
- ½ teaspoon Italian seasoning.

DIRECTIONS:

1. Preheat the air fryer to 360°F.
2. Peel the eggplants and chop them.
3. Put the chopped eggplants in the air fryer basket.
4. Chop the cherry tomatoes and add them to the air fryer basket.
5. Then add chopped onion, sliced garlic clove, olive oil, ground black pepper, and Italian seasoning.
6. Chop the sweet yellow pepper roughly and add it to the air fryer basket.
7. Shake the vegetables gently and cook for 15 minutes.
8. Stir the meal after 8 minutes of cooking.
9. Transfer the cooked ratatouille to the serving plates.
10. Enjoy!

NUTRITION:

- Calories: 149.
- Fat: 3.7 g.
- Fiber: 11.7 g.
- Carbs: 28.9 g.
- Protein: 5.1 g.

- **Cheddar Portobello Mushrooms**

Preparation Time: 15 Minutes.

Cooking Time: 6 Minutes.

Servings: 2.

INGREDIENTS:

- 2 Portobello mushroom hats.
- 2 slices Cheddar cheese.
- ¼ cup panko breadcrumbs.
- ½ teaspoon salt.
- ½ teaspoon ground black pepper.
- 1 egg.
- 1 teaspoon oatmeal.
- 2 oz. bacon, chopped cooked.

DIRECTIONS:

1. Crack the egg into the bowl and whisk it.
2. Combine the ground black pepper, oatmeal, salt, and breadcrumbs in a separate bowl.
3. Dip the mushroom hats in the whisked egg.
4. After this, coat the mushroom hats in the breadcrumb mixture.
5. Preheat the air fryer to 400°F.
6. Place the mushrooms in the air fryer basket tray and cook for 3 minutes.
7. After this, put the chopped bacon and sliced cheese over the mushroom hats, and cook the meal for 3 minutes.
8. When the meal is cooked, let it chill gently.
9. Enjoy!

NUTRITION:

- Calories: 376.
- Fat: 24.1 g.
- Fiber: 1.8 g.
- Carbs: 14.6 g.
- Protein: 25.2 g.

- **Fluffy Bites**

Preparation Time: 20 Minutes.

Cooking Time: 60 Minutes.

Servings: 12.

INGREDIENTS:

- 2 teaspoons cinnamon.
- 2/3 cup sour cream.
- 2 cups heavy cream.
- 1 teaspoon scraped vanilla bean.
- ¼ teaspoon cardamom.
- 4 egg yolks.
- Stevia to taste.

DIRECTIONS:

1. Start by whisking your egg yolks until creamy and smooth.
2. Get out a double boiler, and add your eggs with the rest of your ingredients. Mix well.
3. Remove from heat, allowing it to cool until it reaches room temperature.
4. Refrigerate for an hour before whisking well.
5. Pour into molds, and freeze for at least an hour before serving.

NUTRITION:

- Calories: 363.
- Protein: 2 g.
- Fat: 40 g.
- Carbohydrates: 1 g.

- **Coconut Fudge**

Preparation Time: 20 Minutes.

Cooking Time: 60 Minutes.

Servings: 12.

INGREDIENTS:

- 2 cups coconut oil.
- ½ cup dark cocoa powder.
- ½ cup coconut cream.
- ¼ cup almonds, chopped.
- ¼ cup coconut, shredded.
- 1 teaspoon almond extract.
- Pinch of salt.
- Stevia to taste.

DIRECTIONS:

1. Pour your coconut oil and coconut cream into a bowl, whisking with an electric beater until smooth. Once the mixture becomes smooth and glossy, do not continue.

2. Begin to add in your cocoa powder while mixing slowly, making sure that there aren't any lumps.

3. Add in the rest of your ingredients, and mix well.

4. Line a pan with parchment paper, and freeze until it sets.

5. Slice into squares before serving.

NUTRITION:

- Calories: 172.
- Fat: 20 g.
- Carbohydrates: 3 g.

- **Nutmeg Nougat**

Preparation Time: 30 Minutes.

Cooking Time: 60 Minutes.

Servings: 12.

INGREDIENTS:

- 1 cup heavy cream.
- 1 cup cashew butter.
- 1 cup coconut, shredded.
- ½ teaspoon nutmeg.
- 1 teaspoon vanilla extract, pure.
- Stevia to taste.

DIRECTIONS:

1. Melt your cashew butter using a double boiler, and then stir in your vanilla extract, dairy cream, nutmeg, and stevia. Make sure it's mixed well.

2. Remove from heat, allowing it to cool down before refrigerating it for half an hour.

3. Shape into balls, and coat with shredded coconut. Chill for at least two hours before serving.

NUTRITION:

- Calories: 341.
- Fat: 34 g.
- Carbohydrates: 5 g.

- **Sweet Almond Bites**

Preparation Time: 30 Minutes.

Cooking Time: 90 Minutes.

Servings: 12.

INGREDIENTS:

- 18 ounces butter, grass-fed.
- 2 ounces heavy cream.
- ½ cup Stevia.
- 2/3 cup cocoa powder.
- 1 teaspoon vanilla extract, pure.
- 4 tablespoons almond butter.

DIRECTIONS:

1. Use a double boiler to melt your butter before adding in all of your remaining ingredients.
2. Place the mixture into molds, freezing for two hours before serving.

NUTRITION:

- Calories: 350.
- Protein: 2 g.
- Fat: 38 g.

- **Strawberry Cheesecake Minis**

Preparation Time: 30 Minutes.

Cooking Time: 120 Minutes.

Servings: 5.

INGREDIENTS:

- 1 cup coconut oil.

- 1 cup coconut butter.

- ½ cup strawberries, sliced.

- ½ teaspoon lime juice.

- 2 tablespoons cream cheese, full fat.

- Stevia to taste.

DIRECTIONS:

1. Blend your strawberries together.

2. Soften your cream cheese, and then add in your coconut butter.

3. Combine all ingredients together, and then pour your mixture into silicone molds.

4. Freeze for at least two hours before serving.

NUTRITION:

- Calories: 372.

- Protein: 1 g.

- Fat: 41 g.

- Carbohydrates: 2 g.

- Carbohydrates: 1 g.

- **Cocoa Brownies**

Preparation Time: 10 Minutes.

Cooking Time: 30 Minutes.

Servings: 12.

INGREDIENTS:

- 1 egg.

- 2 tablespoons butter, grass-fed.

- 2 teaspoons vanilla extract, pure.

- ¼ teaspoon baking powder.

- ¼ cup cocoa powder.

- 1/3 cup heavy cream.

- ¾ cup almond butter.

- Pinch sea salt.

DIRECTIONS:

1. Break your egg into a bowl, whisking until smooth.

2. Add in all of your wet ingredients, mixing well.

3. Mix all dry ingredients into a bowl.

4. Sift your dry ingredients into your wet ingredients, mixing to form a batter.

5. Get out a baking pan, greasing it before pouring in your mixture.

6. Heat your oven to 350 and bake for twenty-five minutes.

7. Allow it to cool before slicing and serve at room temperature or warm.

NUTRITION:

- Calories: 184.

- Protein: 1 g.

- Fat: 20 g.

- **Chocolate Orange Bites**

Preparation Time: 20 Minutes.

Cooking Time: 120 Minutes.

Servings: 10.

INGREDIENTS:

- 10 ounces coconut oil.

- 4 tablespoons cocoa powder.

- ¼ teaspoon orange extract.

- Stevia to taste.

DIRECTIONS:

1. Melt half of your coconut oil using a double boiler, and then add in your stevia and orange extract.

2. Get out candy molds, pouring the mixture into it. Fill each mold halfway, and then place in the fridge until they set.

3. Melt the other half of your coconut oil, stirring in your cocoa powder and stevia, making sure that the mixture is smooth with no lumps.

4. Pour into your molds, filling them up all the way, and then allow it to set in the fridge before serving.

NUTRITION:

- Calories: 188.

- Protein: 1 g.

- Fat: 21 g.

- Carbohydrates: 5 g.

- **Caramel Cones**

Preparation Time: 25 Minutes.

Cooking Time: 120 Minutes.

Servings: 5.

INGREDIENTS:

- 2 tablespoons heavy whipping cream.

- 2 tablespoons sour cream.

- 1 tablespoon caramel sugar.

- 1 teaspoon sea salt, fine.

- 1/3 cup butter, grass-fed.

- 1/3 cup coconut oil.

- Stevia to taste.

DIRECTIONS:

1. Soften your coconut oil and butter, mixing together.

2. Mix all ingredients to form a batter, and then place them in molds.

3. Top with a little salt, and keep refrigerated until serving.

NUTRITION:

- Calories: 100.

- Fat: 12 g.

- Carbohydrates: 1 g.

- **Cinnamon Bites**

Preparation Time: 20 Minutes.

Cooking Time: 95 Minutes.

Servings: 5.

INGREDIENTS:

- 1/8 teaspoon nutmeg.
- 1 teaspoon vanilla extract.
- ¼ teaspoon cinnamon.
- 4 tablespoons coconut oil.
- ½ cup butter, grass-fed.
- 8 ounces cream cheese.
- Stevia to taste.

DIRECTIONS:

1. Soften your coconut oil and butter, mixing in your cream cheese.
2. Add all of your remaining ingredients, and mix well.
3. Pour into molds, and freeze until set.

NUTRITION:

- Calories: 178.
- Protein: 1 g.
- Fat: 19 g.

- **Sweet Chai Bites**

Preparation Time: 20 Minutes.

Cooking Time: 45 Minutes.

Servings: 5.

INGREDIENTS:

- 1 cup cream cheese.

- 1 cup coconut oil.

- 2 ounces butter, grass-fed.

- 2 teaspoons ginger.

- 2 teaspoons cardamom.

- 1 teaspoon nutmeg.

- 1 teaspoon cloves.

- 1 teaspoon vanilla extract, pure.

- 1 teaspoon Darjeeling black tea.

- Stevia to taste.

DIRECTIONS:

1. Melt your coconut oil and butter before adding in your black tea. Allow it to set for one to two minutes.

2. Add in your cream cheese, removing your mixture from heat.

3. Add in all of your spices, and stir to combine.

4. Pour into molds, and freeze before serving.

NUTRITION:

- Calories: 178.

- Protein: 1 g.

- Fat: 19 g.

- **Easy Vanilla Bombs**

Preparation Time: 20 Minutes.

Cooking Time: 45 Minutes.

Servings: 12.

INGREDIENTS:

- 1 cup macadamia nuts, unsalted.

- ¼ cup coconut oil.

- ¼ cup butter.

- 2 teaspoons vanilla extract, sugar-free.

- 20 drops liquid Stevia.

- 2 tablespoons erythritol, powdered.

DIRECTIONS::

1. Pulse your macadamia nuts in a blender, and then combine all of your ingredients together. Mix well.

2. Get out mini muffin tins with a tablespoon and a half of the mixture.

3. Refrigerate it for a half-hour before serving.

NUTRITION:

- Calories: 125.

- Fat: 5 g.

- Carbohydrates: 5 g.

- **Marinated Eggs**

Preparation Time: 2 hours, 15 Minutes.

Cooking Time: 7 Minutes.

Servings: 5.

INGREDIENTS:

- 6 eggs.
- 1 and ¼ cups water.
- ¼ cup unsweetened rice vinegar.
- 2 tablespoons coconut aminos.
- Salt and black pepper to the taste.
- 2 garlic cloves, minced.
- 1 teaspoon stevia.
- 4 ounces cream cheese.
- 1 tablespoon chives.

DIRECTIONS:

1. Put the eggs in a pot, add water to cover, bring to a boil over medium heat, cover and cook for 7 minutes.
2. Rinse eggs with cold water and leave them aside to cool down.
3. In a bowl, mix one cup of water with coconut aminos, vinegar, stevia, and garlic and whisk well.
4. Put the eggs in this mix, cover with a kitchen towel, and leave them aside for 2 hours, rotating from time to time.
5. Peel eggs, cut in halves and put egg yolks in a bowl.
6. Add ¼ cup water, cream cheese, salt, pepper, and chives and stir well.
7. Stuff egg whites with this mix and serve them.
8. Enjoy!

NUTRITION:

- Calories: 289.
- Protein: 15.86 g.
- Fat: 22.62 g.
- Carbohydrates: 4.52 g.
- Sodium: 288 mg.

- **Cheesy Mashed Cauliflower with Bacon**

Preparation Time: 10 Minutes.

Cooking Time: 40 Minutes.

Servings: 6.

INGREDIENTS:

- 6 slices bacon.

- 2 heads cauliflower, chopped.

- 2 cups water.

- 2 tbsp butter, melted.

- ½ cup buttermilk Salt and black pepper to taste.

- ¼ cup yellow cheddar cheese, grated.

- 2 tbsp chopped chives.

DIRECTIONS:

1. Preheat oven to 350°F.

2. Fry bacon in a heated skillet over medium heat for 5 minutes until crispy. Remove to a paper towel-lined plate, allow to cool, and crumble. Set aside and keep bacon fat.

3. Boil the cauliflower in water in a pot over high heat for 7 minutes until tender. Drain and put in a bowl. Include butter, buttermilk, salt, and pepper, and puree using a hand blender until smooth and creamy.

4. Lightly grease a casserole dish with the bacon fat and spread the mash on it. Sprinkle with cheddar cheese and place under the broiler for 4 minutes on high until the cheese melts. Remove and top with bacon and chopped chives.

5. Serve with pan-seared scallops.

NUTRITION:

- Calories: 132.

- Protein: 6.79 g.

- Fat: 9.58 g.

- Carbohydrates: 6.22 g.

- Sodium: 362 mg.

- **Tasty Onion and Cauliflower Dip**

Preparation Time: 20 Minutes.

Cooking Time: 30 Minutes.

Servings: 15.

INGREDIENTS:

- 1 and ½ cups chicken stock.
- 1 cauliflower head, florets separated.
- ¼ cup mayonnaise.
- ½ cup yellow onion, chopped.
- ¾ cup cream cheese.
- ½ teaspoon chili powder.
- ½ teaspoon cumin, ground.
- ½ teaspoon garlic powder.
- Salt and black pepper to the taste.

DIRECTIONS:

1. Put the stock in a pot, add cauliflower and onion, heat up over medium heat, and cook for 30 minutes.
2. Add chili powder, salt, pepper, cumin, and garlic powder and stir.
3. Also, add cream cheese and stir a bit until it melts.
4. Blend using an immersion blender and mix with the mayo.
5. Transfer to a bowl and keep in the fridge for 2 hours before you serve it.
6. Enjoy!

NUTRITION:

- Calories: 40.
- Protein: 1.23 g.
- Fat: 3.31 g.
- Carbohydrates: 1.66 g.
- Sodium: 72 mg.

- **Cheesy Chicken Fritters with Dill Dip**

Preparation Time: 10 Minutes.

Cooking Time: 40 Minutes.

Servings: 5.

INGREDIENTS:

- 1 lb. chicken breasts, thinly sliced.

- 1 ¼ cups mayonnaise.

- ¼ cup coconut flour 2 eggs.

- Salt and black pepper to taste.

- 1 cup mozzarella cheese, grated.

- 2 tbsp. dill, chopped.

- 2 tbsp. olive oil 1 cup sour cream.

- ½ tsp. garlic powder.

- 1 tbsp. parsley, chopped.

- 1 onion, finely chopped.

DIRECTIONS:

1. In a bowl, mix 1 cup of the mayonnaise, dill, sour cream, garlic powder, onion, and salt. Keep in the fridge.

2. Mix the remaining mayonnaise, coconut flour, eggs, salt, pepper, and mozzarella cheese in a bowl. Add in the chicken and toss to coat.

3. Cover the bowl with plastic wrap and refrigerate it for 2 hours.

4. Place a skillet over medium fire and heat the olive oil. Fetch 2 tablespoons of chicken mixture into the skillet, use the back of a spatula to flatten the top. Cook for 4 minutes, flip, and fry for 4 more.

5. Remove onto a wire rack and repeat the cooking process until the chicken ingredients are finished, adding more oil as needed.

6. Garnish the fritters with parsley and serve with the dill dip.

NUTRITION:

- Calories: 9.

- Protein: 0.41 g.

- Fat: 0.14 g.

- Carbohydrates: 1.86 g.

- Sodium: 2 mg.

- **Layered Zucchini & Bell Pepper Bake**

Preparation Time: 10 Minutes.

Cooking Time: 65 Minutes.

Servings: 6.

INGREDIENTS:

- 2 lb. zucchinis, sliced.
- 2 red bell peppers, seeded and sliced.
- Salt and black pepper to taste.
- 1 ½ cups feta cheese, crumbled.
- 2 tbsp. butter, melted.
- ¼ tsp. xanthan gum.
- ½ cup heavy whipping cream.
- 2 tbsp. fresh dill, chopped.

DIRECTIONS:

1. Preheat oven to 370°F. Place the sliced zucchinis in a colander over the sink, sprinkle with salt and let sit for 20 minutes.

2. Transfer to paper towels to drain the excess liquid.

3. Grease a baking dish with cooking spray and make a layer of zucchini and bell peppers overlapping.

4. Season with pepper, and sprinkle with feta cheese. Repeat the layering process a second time.

5. Combine the butter, xanthan gum, salt, and whipping cream in a bowl. Stir to mix completely and pour over the vegetables.

6. Bake for 30–40 minutes or until golden brown on top.

7. Serve sprinkled with dill.

NUTRITION:

- Calories: 65.
- Protein: 2.82 g.
- Fat: 5.42 g.
- Carbohydrates: 2.27 g.
- Sodium: 57 mg.

- **Avocado Dip**

Preparation Time: 5 minutes.

Cooking Time: 0 minutes.

Servings: 8.

INGREDIENTS:

- ½ cup heavy cream.
- 1 green chili pepper, chopped.
- Salt and pepper to the taste.
- 4 avocados, pitted, peeled, and chopped.
- 1 cup cilantro, chopped.
- ¼ cup lime juice.

DIRECTIONS:

1. Pour the cream with the avocados and the rest of the ingredients in a blender, and pulse well.
2. Divide the mix into bowls and serve cold as a party dip.

NUTRITION:

- Calories: 200.
- Fat: 14.5 g.
- Fiber: 3.8 g.
- Carbs: 8.1 g.
- Protein: 7.6 g.

1. Add all ingredients into the inner pot of the instant pot and set the pot on sauté mode.

2. Seal pot with lid and cook on high for 20 minutes.

3. Once done, release pressure using quick release. Remove lid.

4. Shred the meat using a fork.

5. Stir well and serve.

NUTRITION:

- Calories: 456. - Fat: 32.7 g.
- Carbohydrates: 7.7 g.
- Sugar: 4.1 g.
- Protein: 31 g.
- Cholesterol: 118 mg.

BEEF & LAMB

- **Moist Shredded Beef**

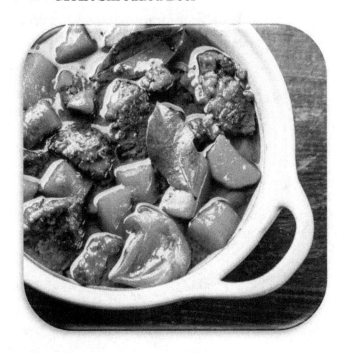

Preparation Time: 10 minutes.

Cooking Time: 20 minutes.

Servings: 8.

INGREDIENTS:

- 2 lbs. beef chuck roast, cut into chunks.
- 1/2 tbsp. dried red pepper.
- 1 tbsp. Italian seasoning.
- 1 tbsp garlic, minced.
- 2 tbsp. vinegar.
- 14 oz. can fire-roasted tomatoes.
- 1/2 cup bell pepper, chopped.
- 1/2 cup carrots, chopped.
- 1 cup onion, chopped.
- 1 tsp. salt.

DIRECTIONS:

- **Hearty Beef Ragu**

Preparation Time: 10 minutes.

Cooking Time: 50 minutes.

Servings: 4.

INGREDIENTS:

- 1 1/2 lbs. beef steak, diced.
- 1 1/2 cup beef stock.
- 1 tbsp. coconut amino.
- 14 oz. can tomatoes, chopped.
- 1/2 tsp. ground cinnamon.
- 1 tsp dried thyme.
- 1 tsp. dried basil.
- 1 tsp. paprika.
- 1 bay leaf.
- 1 tbsp. garlic, chopped.
- 1/2 tsp. cayenne pepper.
- 1 celery stick, diced.
- 1 carrot, diced.
- 1 onion, diced.
- 2 tbsp. olive oil.
- 1/4 tsp. pepper.
- 1 1/2 tsp. sea salt.

DIRECTIONS:

1. Add oil into the instant pot and set the pot on sauté mode.
2. Add celery, carrots, onion, and salt and sauté for 5 minutes.
3. Add meat and remaining ingredients and stir everything well.
4. Seal pot with lid and cook on high for 30 minutes.
5. Once done, allow to release pressure naturally for 10 minutes, then release remaining using quick release. Remove lid.
6. Shred meat using a fork. Set pot on sauté mode and cook for 10 minutes. Stir every 2–3 minutes.
7. Serve and enjoy.

NUTRITION:

- Calories: 435.
- Fat: 18.1 g.
- Carbohydrates: 12.3 g.
- Sugar: 5.5 g.
- Protein: 54.4 g.
- Cholesterol: 152 mg.

- **Dill Beef Brisket**

Preparation Time: 10 minutes.

Cooking Time: 50 minutes.

Servings: 4.

INGREDIENTS:

- 2 1/2 lbs. beef brisket, cut into cubes.
- 2 1/2 cups beef stock.
- 2 tbsp. dill, chopped.
- 1 celery stalk, chopped.
- 1 onion, sliced.
- 1 tbsp. garlic, minced.
- Pepper.
- Salt.

DIRECTIONS:

1. Add all ingredients into the inner pot of the instant pot and stir well.
2. Seal pot with lid and cook on high for 50 minutes.
3. Once done, allow to release pressure naturally for 10 minutes, then release remaining using quick release. Remove lid.
4. Serve and enjoy.

NUTRITION:

- Calories: 556.
- Fat: 18.1 g.
- Carbohydrates: 4.3 g.
- Sugar: 1.3 g.
- Protein: 88.5 g.
- Cholesterol: 253 mg.

- **Tasty Beef Stew**

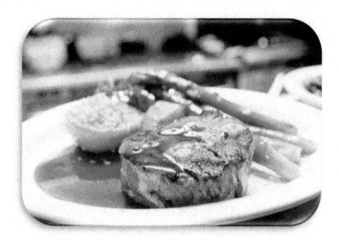

NUTRITION:

- Calories: 562.
- Fat: 18.1 g.
- Carbohydrates: 5.7 g.
- Sugar: 4.6 g.
- Protein: 87.4 g.
- Cholesterol: 253 mg.

Preparation Time: 10 minutes.

Cooking Time: 30 minutes.

Servings: 4.

INGREDIENTS:

- 2 1/2 lbs. beef roast, cut into chunks.
- 1 cup beef broth.
- 1/2 cup balsamic vinegar.
- 1 tbsp. honey.
- 1/2 tsp. red pepper flakes.
- 1 tbsp. garlic, minced.
- Pepper.
- Salt.

DIRECTIONS:

1. Add all ingredients into the inner pot of the instant pot and stir well.
2. Seal pot with lid and cook on high for 30 minutes.
3. Once done, allow to release pressure naturally. Remove lid.
4. Stir well and serve.

- **Meatloaf**

Preparation Time: 10 minutes.

Cooking Time: 35 minutes.

Servings: 6.

INGREDIENTS:

- 2 lbs. ground beef.
- 2 eggs, lightly beaten.
- 1/4 tsp. dried basil.
- 3 tbsp. olive oil.
- 1/2 tsp. dried sage.
- 1 1/2 tsp. dried parsley.
- 1 tsp. oregano.
- 2 tsp. thyme.
- 1 tsp. rosemary.
- Pepper.
- Salt.

NUTRITION:

- Calories: 365.
- Fat: 18 g.
- Carbohydrates: 0.7 g.
- Sugar: 0.1 g.
- Protein: 47.8 g.
- Cholesterol: 190 mg.

DIRECTIONS:

1. Pour 1 1/2 cups of water into the instant pot, then place the trivet in the pot.
2. Spray loaf pan with cooking spray.
3. Add all ingredients into the mixing bowl and mix until well combined.
4. Transfer meat mixture into the prepared loaf pan and place loaf pan on top of the trivet in the pot.
5. Seal pot with lid and cook on high for 35 minutes.
6. Once done, allow to release pressure naturally for 10 minutes, then release remaining using quick release. Remove lid.
7. Serve and enjoy.

- **Flavorful Beef Bourguignon**

Preparation Time: 10 minutes.

Cooking Time: 20 minutes.

Servings: 4.

INGREDIENTS:

- 1 1/2 lbs. beef chuck roast, cut into chunks.
- 2/3 cup beef stock.
- 2 tbsp. fresh thyme.
- 1 bay leaf.
- 1 tsp. garlic, minced.
- 8 oz. mushrooms, sliced.
- 2 tbsp. tomato paste.
- 2/3 cup dry red wine.
- 1 onion, sliced.
- 4 carrots, cut into chunks.
- 1 tbsp. olive oil.
- Pepper.
- Salt.

DIRECTIONS:

1. Add oil into the instant pot and set the pot on sauté mode.
2. Add meat and sauté until brown. Add onion and sauté until softened.
3. Add remaining ingredients and stir well.
4. Seal pot with lid and cook on high for 12 minutes.
5. Once done, allow to release pressure naturally. Remove lid.
6. Stir well and serve.

NUTRITION:

- Calories: 744.
- Fat: 51.3 g.
- Carbohydrates: 14.5 g.
- Sugar: 6.5 g.
- Protein: 48.1 g.
- Cholesterol: 175 mg.

- **Delicious Beef Chili**

Preparation Time: 10 minutes.

Cooking Time: 35 minutes.

Servings: 8.

INGREDIENTS:

- 2 lbs. ground beef.
- 1 tsp. olive oil.
- 1 tsp. garlic, minced.
- 1 small onion, chopped.
- 2 tbsp. chili powder.
- 1 tsp. oregano.
- 1/2 tsp. thyme.
- 28 oz. can tomatoes, crushed.
- 2 cups beef stock.
- 2 carrots, chopped.
- 3 sweet potatoes, peeled and cubed.
- Pepper.
- Salt.

DIRECTIONS:

1. Add oil into the instant pot and set the pot on sauté mode.
2. Add meat and cook until brown.
3. Add remaining ingredients and stir well.
4. Seal pot with lid and cook on high for 35 minutes.
5. Once done, allow to release pressure naturally. Remove lid.
6. Stir well and serve.

NUTRITION:

- Calories: 302.
- Fat: 8.2 g.
- Carbohydrates: 19.2 g.
- Sugar: 4.8 g.
- Protein: 37.1 g.
- Cholesterol: 101 mg.

- **Rosemary Creamy Beef**

Preparation Time: 10 minutes.

Cooking Time: 40 minutes.

Servings: 4.

INGREDIENTS:

- 2 lbs. beef stew meat, cubed.
- 2 tbsp. fresh parsley, chopped.
- 1 tsp. garlic, minced.
- 1/2 tsp. dried rosemary.
- 1 tsp. chili powder.
- 1 cup beef stock.
- 1 cup heavy cream.
- 1 onion, chopped.
- 1 tbsp. olive oil.
- Pepper.
- Salt.

DIRECTIONS:

1. Add oil into the instant pot and set the pot on sauté mode.
2. Add rosemary, garlic, onion, and chili powder and sauté for 5 minutes.
3. Add meat and cook for 5 minutes.
4. Add remaining ingredients and stir well.
5. Seal pot with lid and cook on high for 30 minutes.
6. Once done, allow to release pressure naturally for 10 minutes, then release remaining using quick release. Remove lid.
7. Serve and enjoy.

NUTRITION:

- Calories: 574.
- Fat: 29 g.
- Carbohydrates: 4.3 g.
- Sugar: 1.3 g.
- Protein: 70.6 g.
- Cholesterol: 244 mg.

- **Spicy Beef Chili Verde**

Preparation Time: 10 minutes.

Cooking Time: 23 minutes.

Servings: 2.

INGREDIENTS:

- 1/2 lb. beef stew meat, cut into cubes.
- 1/4 tsp. chili powder.
- 1 tbsp. olive oil.
- 1 cup chicken broth.
- 1 Serrano pepper, chopped.
- 1 tsp. garlic, minced.
- 1 small onion, chopped.
- 1/4 cup grape tomatoes, chopped.
- 1/4 cup tomatillos, chopped.
- Pepper.
- Salt.

DIRECTIONS:

1. Add oil into the instant pot and set the pot on sauté mode.
2. Add garlic and onion and sauté for 3 minutes.
3. Add remaining ingredients and stir well.
4. Seal pot with lid and cook on high for 20 minutes.
5. Once done, allow to release pressure naturally. Remove lid.
6. Stir well and serve.

NUTRITION:

- Calories: 317.
- Fat: 15.1 g.
- Carbohydrates: 6.4 g.
- Sugar: 2.6 g.
- Protein: 37.8 g.
- Cholesterol: 101 mg.

- **Carrot Mushroom Beef Roast**

Preparation Time: 10 minutes.

Cooking Time: 40 minutes.

Servings: 4.

INGREDIENTS:

- 1 1/2 lbs. beef roast.

- 1 tsp. paprika.

- 1/4 tsp. dried rosemary.

- 1 tsp. garlic, minced.

- 1/2 lb. mushrooms, sliced.

- 1/2 cup chicken stock.

- 2 carrots, sliced.

- Pepper.

- Salt.

DIRECTIONS:

1. Add all ingredients into the inner pot of the instant pot and stir well.

2. Seal pot with lid and cook on high for 40 minutes.

3. Once done, allow to release pressure naturally for 10 minutes, then release remaining using quick release. Remove lid.

4. Slice and serve.

NUTRITION:

- Calories: 345.

- Fat: 10.9 g.

- Carbohydrates: 5.6 g.

- Sugar: 2.6 g.

- Protein: 53.8 g.

- Cholesterol: 152 mg.

- **Tender Lamb Chops**

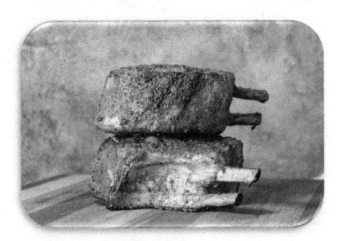

- Calories: 40.
- Fat: 1.9 g.
- Carbohydrates: 2.3 g.
- Sugar: 0.6 g.
- Protein: 3.4 g.
- Cholesterol: 0 mg.

Preparation Time: 10 minutes.

Cooking Time: 6 hours.

Servings: 8.

INGREDIENTS:

- 8 lamb chops.
- ½ teaspoon dried thyme.
- 1 onion, sliced.
- 1 teaspoon dried oregano.
- 2 garlic cloves, minced.
- Pepper and salt.

DIRECTIONS:

1. Add sliced onion into the slow cooker.
2. Combine together thyme, oregano, pepper, and salt. Rub over lamb chops.
3. Place lamb chops in the slow cooker and top with garlic.
4. Pour ¼ cup water around the lamb chops.
5. Cover and cook on low heat for 6 hours.
6. Serve and enjoy.

NUTRITION:

- **Beef Stroganoff**

Preparation Time: 10 minutes.

Cooking Time: 8 hours.

Servings: 2.

INGREDIENTS:

- 1/2 lb beef stew meat.
- 10 oz mushroom soup, homemade.
- 1 medium onion, chopped.
- 1/2 cup sour cream.
- 2.5 oz mushrooms, sliced.
- Pepper and salt.

DIRECTIONS:

1. Add all ingredients except sour cream into the crockpot and mix well.
2. Cover and cook on low heat for 8 hours.
3. Add sour cream and stir well.
4. Serve and enjoy.

NUTRITION:

- Calories: 470.
- Fat: 25 g.
- Carbohydrates: 8.6 g.
- Sugar: 3 g.
- Protein: 49 g.
- Cholesterol: 108 mg.

- **Lemon Beef**

Preparation Time: 10 minutes.

Cooking Time: 6 hours.

Servings: 4.

INGREDIENTS:

- 1 lb beef chuck roast.
- 1 fresh lime juice.
- 1 garlic clove, crushed.
- 1 teaspoon chili powder.
- 2 cups lemon-lime soda.
- 1/2 teaspoon salt.

DIRECTIONS:

1. Place beef chuck roast into the slow cooker.
2. Season roast with garlic, chili powder, and salt.
3. Pour lemon-lime soda over the roast.
4. Cover slow cooker and cook on low for 6 hours. Shred the meat using a fork.
5. Add lime juice over shredded roast and serve.

NUTRITION:

- Calories: 355.
- Fat: 16.8 g.
- Carbohydrates: 14 g.
- Sugar: 11.3 g.
- Protein: 35.5 g.
- Cholesterol: 120 mg.

- **Greek Beef Roast**

Preparation Time: 10 minutes.

Cooking Time: 8 hours.

Servings: 6.

INGREDIENTS:

- 2 lbs lean top round beef roast.
- 1 tablespoon Italian seasoning.
- 6 garlic cloves, minced.
- 1 onion, sliced.
- 2 cups beef broth.
- ½ cup red wine.
- 1 teaspoon red pepper flakes.
- Pepper.
- Salt.

DIRECTIONS:

1. Season meat with pepper and salt and place into the crockpot.
2. Pour remaining ingredients over meat.
3. Cover and cook on low heat for 8 hours.
4. Shred the meat using a fork.
5. Serve and enjoy.

NUTRITION:

- Calories: 231.
- Fat: 6 g.
- Carbohydrates: 4 g.
- Sugar: 1.4 g.
- Protein: 35 g.
- Cholesterol: 75 mg.

- **Moroccan Meatballs**

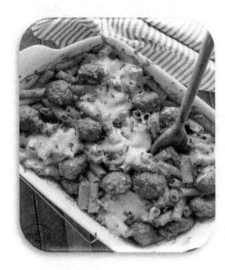

Preparation Time: 10 Minutes.

Cooking Time: 20 Minutes.

Servings: 5.

INGREDIENTS:

- ¼ cup finely chopped onion (about ⅛ onion).
- ¼ cup raisins, coarsely chopped.
- 1 teaspoon ground cumin.
- ½ teaspoon ground cinnamon.
- ¼ teaspoon smoked paprika.
- 1 large egg.
- 1 pound ground beef (93% lean) or ground lamb.
- ⅓ cup panko bread crumbs.
- 1 teaspoon extra-virgin olive oil.
- 1 (28-ounce) can low-sodium or no-salt-added crushed tomatoes Chopped fresh mint, feta cheese, and/or fresh orange or lemon wedges, for serving.

DIRECTIONS:

1. In a large bowl, combine the onion, raisins, cumin, cinnamon, smoked paprika, and egg. Add the ground beef and bread crumbs and mix gently with your hands. Divide the mixture into 20 even portions, then wet your hands and roll each portion into a ball. Wash your hands.

2. In a large skillet over medium-high heat, heat the oil. Add the meatballs and cook for 8 minutes, rolling around every minute or so with tongs or a fork to brown them on most sides. (They won't be cooked through.) Transfer the meatballs to a paper towel-lined plate. Drain the fat out of the pan, and carefully wipe out the hot pan with a paper towel.

3. Return the meatballs to the pan, and pour the tomatoes over the meatballs. Cover and cook on medium-high heat until the sauce begins to bubble. Lower the heat to medium, cover partially, and cook for 7 to 8 more minutes, until the meatballs are cooked through. Garnish with fresh mint, feta cheese, and/or a squeeze of citrus, if desired, and serve.

NUTRITION:

- Calories: 306. - Total Fat: 10 g.
- Saturated Fat: 4 g.
- Cholesterol: 117 mg.
- Sodium: 342 mg.
- Total Carbohydrates: 26 g.
- Fiber: 7 g. - Protein: 29 g.

- **Beef Spanakopita Pita Pockets**

Preparation Time: 5 Minutes.

Cooking Time: 15 Minutes.

Servings: 5.

INGREDIENTS:

- 3 teaspoons extra-virgin olive oil, divided.

- 1 pound ground beef (93% lean).

- 2 garlic cloves, minced.

- 2 (6-ounce) bags baby spinach, chopped.

- ½ cup crumbled feta cheese (about 2 ounces).

- ⅓ cup ricotta cheese.

- ½ teaspoon ground nutmeg.

- ¼ teaspoon freshly ground black pepper.

- ¼ cup slivered almonds.

- 4 (6-inch) whole-wheat pita breads, cut in half.

DIRECTIONS:

1. In a large skillet over medium heat, heat 1 teaspoon of oil. Add the ground beef and cook for 10 minutes, breaking it up with a wooden spoon and stirring occasionally. Remove from the heat and drain in a colander. Set the meat aside.

2. Place the skillet back on the heat, and add the remaining 2 teaspoons of oil. Add the garlic and cook for 1 minute, stirring constantly. Add the spinach and cook for 2 to 3 minutes, or until the spinach has cooked down, stirring often.

3. Turn off the heat and mix in the feta cheese, ricotta, nutmeg, and pepper. Stir until all the ingredients are well incorporated. Mix in the almonds.

4. Divide the beef filling among the eight pita pocket halves to stuff them and serve.

NUTRITION:

- Calories: 506.

- Total Fat: 22 g.

- Saturated Fat: 8 g.

- Cholesterol: 98 mg.

- Sodium: 567 mg.

- Total Carbohydrates: 42 g.

- Fiber: 8 g.

- Protein: 39 g.

- ## Grilled Steak, Mushroom, and Onion Kebabs

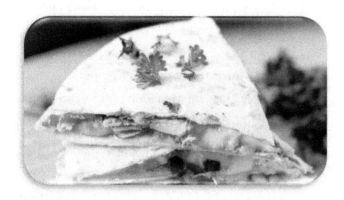

Preparation Time: 15 Minutes.

Cooking Time: 15 Minutes.

Servings: 5.

INGREDIENTS:

- Non-stick cooking spray.
- 4 garlic cloves, peeled.
- 2 fresh rosemary sprigs (about 3 inches each).
- 2 tablespoons extra-virgin olive oil, divided.
- 1 pound boneless top sirloin steak, about 1 inch thick 1 (8-ounce) package white button mushrooms.
- 1 medium red onion, cut into 12 thin wedges.
- ¼ teaspoon coarsely ground black pepper.
- 2 tablespoons red wine vinegar.
- ¼ teaspoon kosher or sea salt.

DIRECTIONS:

1. Soak 12 (10-inch) wooden skewers in water. Spray the cold grill with non-stick cooking spray, and heat the grill to medium-high.

2. Cut a piece of aluminum foil into a 10-inch square. Place the garlic and rosemary sprigs in the center, drizzle with 1 tablespoon of oil, and wrap tightly to form a foil packet. Place it on the grill, and close the grill cover.

3. Cut the steak into 1-inch cubes. Thread the beef onto the wet skewers, alternating with whole mushrooms and onion wedges. Spray the kebabs thoroughly with non-stick cooking spray, and sprinkle with pepper.

4. Cook the kebabs on the covered grill for 4 to 5 minutes. Turn and grill 4 to 5 more minutes, covered, until a meat thermometer inserted in the meat registers 145°F (medium rare) or 160°F (medium).

5. Remove the foil packet from the grill, open, and, using tongs, place the garlic and rosemary sprigs in a small bowl. Carefully strip the rosemary sprigs of their leaves into the bowl and pour in any accumulated juices and oil from the foil packet. Add the remaining 1 tablespoon of oil and the vinegar and salt. Mash the garlic with a fork, and mix all ingredients in the bowl together. Pour over the finished steak kebabs and serve.

NUTRITION:

- Calories: 300.
- Total Fat: 14 g.
- Saturated Fat: 4 g.
- Cholesterol: 101 mg.
- Sodium: 196 mg.
- Total Carbohydrates: 6 g.
- Fiber: 1 g.
- Protein: 36 g.

- **Beef Gyros with Tahini Sauce**

Preparation Time: 15 Minutes.

Cooking Time: 10 Minutes.

Servings: 5.

INGREDIENTS:

- Non-stick cooking spray.

- 2 tablespoons extra-virgin olive oil.

- 1 tablespoon dried oregano.

- 1 ¼ teaspoon garlic powder, divided.

- 1 teaspoon ground cumin.

- ½ teaspoon freshly ground black pepper.

- ¼ teaspoon kosher or sea salt.

- 1 pound beef flank steak, top round steak, or lamb leg steak, center cut, about 1 inch thick.

- 1 medium green bell pepper, halved and seeded.

- 2 tablespoons tahini or peanut butter.

- 1 tablespoon hot water.

- ½ cup 2% plain Greek yogurt.

- 1 tablespoon freshly squeezed lemon juice (about ½ small lemon).

- 1 cup thinly sliced red onion (about ½ onion).

- 4 (6-inch) whole-wheat pita breads, warmed.

DIRECTIONS:

1. Set an oven rack about 4 inches below the broiler element. Preheat the oven broiler to high. Line a large, rimmed baking sheet with foil. Place a wire cooling rack on the foil, and spray the rack with non-stick cooking spray. Set aside.

2. In a small bowl, whisk together the oil, oregano, 1 teaspoon of garlic powder, cumin, pepper, and salt. Rub the oil mixture on all sides of the steak, saving 1 teaspoon of the mixture. Place the steak on the prepared rack. Rub the remaining oil mixture on the bell pepper, and place on the rack, cut-side down. Press the pepper with the heel of your hand to flatten.

3. Broil for 5 minutes. Turn the meat and the pepper pieces, and broil for 2 to 5 more minutes, until the pepper is charred and the internal temperature of the meat measures 145°F on a meat thermometer. Put the pepper and steak on a cutting board to rest for 5 minutes.

4. While the meat is broiling, in a small bowl, whisk the tahini until smooth (adding 1 tablespoon of hot water if your tahini is sticky). Add the remaining ¼ teaspoon of garlic powder and the yogurt and lemon juice, and whisk thoroughly.

5. Slice the steak crosswise into ¼-inch-thick strips. Slice the bell pepper into strips. Divide the steak, bell pepper, and onion among the warm pita breads. Drizzle with tahini sauce and serve.

NUTRITION:

- Calories: 497.

- Total Fat: 21 g.

- Saturated Fat: 5 g.

- Cholesterol: 53 mg.

- Sodium: 548 mg.

- Total Carbohydrates: 45 g.

- Fiber: 7 g.

- Protein: 36 g.

- **Beef Sliders with Pepper Slaw**

Preparation Time: 10 Minutes.

Cooking Time: 10 Minutes.

Servings: 5.

INGREDIENTS:

- Non-stick cooking spray.

- 1 (8-ounce) package white button mushrooms.

- 2 tablespoons extra-virgin olive oil, divided 1 pound ground beef (93% lean).

- 2 garlic cloves, minced (about 1 teaspoon).

- ½ teaspoon kosher or sea salt, divided.

- ¼ teaspoon freshly ground black pepper.

- 1 tablespoon balsamic vinegar.

- 2 bell peppers of different colors, sliced into strips.

- 2 tablespoons torn fresh basil or flat-leaf (Italian) parsley Mini or slider whole-grain rolls, for serving (optional).

DIRECTIONS:

1. Set one oven rack about 4 inches below the broiler element. Preheat the oven broiler to high.

2. Line a large, rimmed baking sheet with aluminum foil. Place a wire cooling rack on the aluminum foil, and spray the rack with non-stick cooking spray. Set aside.

3. Put half the mushrooms in the bowl of a food processor and pulse about 15 times until the mushrooms are finely chopped but not puréed, similar to the texture of ground meat. Repeat with the remaining mushrooms.

4. In a large skillet over medium-high heat, heat 1 tablespoon of oil. Add the mushrooms and cook for 2 to 3 minutes, occasionally stirring, until the mushrooms have cooked down and some of their liquid has evaporated. Remove from the heat.

5. In a large bowl, combine the ground beef with the cooked mushrooms, garlic, ¼ teaspoon of salt, and pepper. Mix gently using your hands. Form the meat into 8 small (½-inch-thick) patties, and place on the prepared rack, making two lines of 4 patties down the center of the pan.

6. .Place the pan in the oven, so the broiler heating element is directly over as many burgers as possible. Broil for 4 minutes. Flip the burgers and rearrange them, so any burgers not getting brown are nearer to the heat source. Broil for 3 to 4 more minutes, or until the internal temperature of the meat is 160°F on a meat thermometer. Watch carefully to prevent burning.

7. While the burgers are cooking, in a large bowl, whisk together the remaining 1 tablespoon of oil, vinegar, and remaining ¼ teaspoon of salt. Add the peppers and basil, and stir gently to coat with the dressing. Serve the sliders with the pepper slaw as a topping or on the side. If desired, serve with the rolls, burger style.

NUTRITION:

- Calories: 259.

- Total Fat: 15 g.

- Saturated Fat: 4 g.

- Cholesterol: 73 mg.

- Sodium: 315 mg.
- Total Carbohydrates: 5 g.
- Fiber: 2 g.
- Protein: 26 g.

- **Mini Greek Meatloaves**

Preparation Time: 5 Minutes.

Cooking Time: 25 Minutes.

Servings: 5.

INGREDIENTS:

- Non-stick cooking spray.
- 1 tablespoon extra-virgin olive oil.
- ½ cup minced onion (about ¼ onion).
- 1 garlic clove, minced (about ½ teaspoon).
- 1 pound ground beef (93% lean).
- ½ cup whole-wheat bread crumbs.
- ½ cup crumbled feta cheese (about 2 ounces).
- 1 large egg.
- ½ teaspoon dried oregano, crushed between your fingers.
- ¼ teaspoon freshly ground black pepper.
- ½ cup 2% plain Greek yogurt.
- ⅓ cup chopped and pitted Kalamata olives.
- 2 tablespoons olive brine.
- Romaine lettuce or pita bread, for serving (optional).

DIRECTIONS:

1. Preheat the oven to 400°F. Coat a 12-cup muffin pan with non-stick cooking spray and set aside.

2. In a small skillet over medium heat, heat the oil. Add the onion and cook for 4 minutes, stirring frequently. Add the garlic and cook for 1 more minute, stirring frequently. Remove from the heat.

3. In a large mixing bowl, combine the onion and garlic with the ground beef, bread crumbs, feta, egg, oregano, and pepper. Gently mix together with your hands.

4. Divide into 12 portions and place in the muffin cups. Cook for 18 to 20 minutes, or until the internal temperature of the meat is 160°F on a meat thermometer.

5. While the meatloaves are baking, in a small bowl, whisk together the yogurt, olives, and olive brine.

6. When you're ready to serve, place the meatloaves on a serving platter and spoon the olive-yogurt sauce on top. You can also serve them on a bed of lettuce or with cut-up pieces of pita bread.

NUTRITION:

- Calories: 244.
- Total Fat: 13 g.
- Saturated Fat: 5 g.
- Cholesterol: 87 mg.
- Sodium: 355 mg.
- Total Carbohydrates: 10 g.
- Fiber: 1 g.
- Protein: 22g.

PORK

- **Smoky Pork & Cabbage**

Preparation Time: 15 Minutes.

Cooking Time: 8 hours.

Servings: 5.

INGREDIENTS:

- 3 lbs. pork roast.
- 1/2 cabbage head, chopped.
- 1 cup water.
- 1/3 cup liquid smoke.
- 1 tablespoon kosher salt.

DIRECTIONS:

1. Rub pork with kosher salt and place into the crockpot.
2. Pour liquid smoke over the pork. Add water.
3. Cover and cook on low heat for 7 hours.
4. Remove pork from the crockpot and add cabbage to the bottom of the crockpot.
5. Place pork on top of the cabbage.
6. Cover again and cook for 1 more hour.
7. Shred pork with a fork and serve.

NUTRITION:

- Calories: 484.
- Fat: 21.5 g.
- Carbohydrates: 4 g.
- Sugar: 1.9 g.
- Protein: 66 g.
- Cholesterol: 195 mg.

- **Seasoned Pork Chops**

Preparation Time: 15 Minutes.

Cooking Time: 4 hours.

Servings: 5.

INGREDIENTS:

- 4 pork chops.

- 2 garlic cloves, minced.

- 1 cup chicken broth.

- 1 tablespoon poultry seasoning.

- 1/4 cup olive oil.

- Pepper and salt.

DIRECTIONS:

1. In a bowl, whisk together olive oil, poultry seasoning, garlic, broth, pepper, and salt.

2. Pour olive oil mixture into the slow cooker, then place pork chops in the crockpot.

3. Cover and cook on high heat for 4 hours.

4. Serve and enjoy.

NUTRITION:

- Calories: 324.

- Fat: 2 g.

- Carbs: 6 g.

- Protein: 6 g.

- Sodium: 344 g.

- **Herb Pork Roast**

Preparation Time: 15 Minutes.

Cooking Time: 8 hours.

Servings: 5.

INGREDIENTS:

- 5 lbs pork roast, boneless or bone-in.
- 1 tablespoon dry herb mix.
- 4 garlic cloves, cut into slivers.
- 1 tablespoon salt.

DIRECTIONS:

1. Using a knife, make small cuts all over the meat, then insert garlic slivers into the cuts.
2. In a small bowl, mix together Italian herb mix and salt and rub all over pork roast.
3. Place pork roast in the crockpot.
4. Cover and cook on low heat for 14 hours.
5. Extract meat from crockpot and shred using a fork.
6. Serve and enjoy.

NUTRITION:

- Calories: 327.
- Fat: 8 g.
- Carbohydrates: 0.5 g.
- Sugar: 0 g.
- Protein: 59 g.
- Cholesterol: 166 mg.

- **Tomato Pork Chops**

Preparation Time: 15 Minutes.

Cooking Time: 6 hours.

Servings: 5.

INGREDIENTS:

- 4 pork chops, bone-in.

- 1 tablespoon garlic, minced.

- ½ small onion, chopped.

- 6 oz. can tomato paste.

- 1 bell pepper, chopped.

- ¼ teaspoon red pepper flakes.

- 1 teaspoon Worcestershire sauce.

- 1 tablespoon dried Italian seasoning.

- 1 oz can tomatoes, diced.

- 2 teaspoon olive oil.

- ¼ teaspoon pepper.

- 1 teaspoon kosher salt.

DIRECTIONS:

1. Heat oil in a pan over heat.

2. Season pork chops with pepper and salt.

3. Sear pork chops in a pan until brown from both sides.

4. Transfer pork chops into the crockpot.

5. Add remaining ingredients over pork chops.

6. Cover and cook on low heat for 6 hours.

7. Serve and enjoy.

NUTRITION:

- Calories: 325.

- Fat: 23.4 g.

- Carbohydrates: 10 g.

- Sugar: 6 g.

- Protein: 20 g.

- Cholesterol: 70 mg.

- **Greek Pork Chops**

Preparation Time: 15 Minutes.

Cooking Time: 6 Minutes.

Servings: 5.

INGREDIENTS:

- 8 pork chops, boneless.
- 4 teaspoon dried oregano.
- 2 tablespoon Worcestershire sauce.
- 3 tablespoon fresh lemon juice.
- ¼ cup olive oil.
- 1 teaspoon ground mustard.
- 2 teaspoon garlic powder.
- 2 teaspoon onion powder.
- Pepper.
- Salt.

DIRECTIONS:

1. Whisk together oil, garlic powder, onion powder, oregano, Worcestershire sauce, lemon juice, mustard, pepper, and salt.
2. Place pork chops in a dish, then pour marinade over pork chops and coat well. Place in refrigerator overnight.
3. Preheat the grill.
4. Place pork chops on the grill and cook for 3–4 minutes on each side.
5. Serve and enjoy.

NUTRITION:

- Calories: 324.
- Fat: 26.5 g.
- Carbohydrates: 2.5 g.
- Sugar: 1.3 g.
- Protein: 18 g.
- Cholesterol: 69 mg.

- **Pork Cacciatore**

Preparation Time: 15 Minutes.

Cooking Time: 6 hours.

Servings: 5.

INGREDIENTS:

- 1 ½ lbs. pork chops.
- 1 teaspoon dried oregano.
- 1 cup beef broth.
- 3 tablespoon tomato paste.
- 14 oz. can tomatoes, diced.
- 2 cups mushrooms, sliced.
- 1 small onion, diced.
- 1 garlic clove, minced.
- 2 tablespoon olive oil.
- ¼ teaspoon pepper.
- ½ teaspoon salt.

DIRECTIONS:

1. Heat oil in a pan over medium heat.
2. Add pork chops in a pan and cook until brown on both sides.
3. Transfer pork chops into the crockpot.
4. Pour remaining ingredients over the pork chops.
5. Cover and cook on low heat for 6 hours.
6. Serve and enjoy.

NUTRITION:

- Calories: 440.
- Fat: 33 g.
- Carbohydrates: 6 g.
- Sugar: 3 g.
- Protein: 28 g.
- Cholesterol: 97 mg.

- **Pork Roast**

Preparation Time: 15 Minutes.

Cooking Time: 1 hour.

Servings: 5.

INGREDIENTS:

- 3 lbs. pork roast, boneless.
- 1 cup water.
- 1 onion, chopped.
- 3 garlic cloves, chopped.
- 1 tablespoon black pepper.
- 1 rosemary sprig.
- 2 fresh oregano sprigs.
- 2 fresh thyme sprigs.
- 1 tablespoon olive oil.
- 1 tablespoon kosher salt.

DIRECTIONS:

1. Preheat the oven to 350°F.
2. Season pork roast with pepper and salt.
3. Add onion and garlic. Pour in the water, oregano, and thyme and bring to boil for a minute.
4. Cover pot and roast in the preheated oven for 1 1/2 hours.
5. Serve and enjoy.

NUTRITION:

- Calories: 502.
- Fat: 23.8 g.
- Carbohydrates: 3 g.
- Sugar: 0.8 g.
- Protein: 65 g.
- Cholesterol: 195 mg.

- **Lemon Pepper Pork Tenderloin**

Preparation Time: 15 Minutes.

Cooking Time: 25 Minutes.

Servings: 5.

INGREDIENTS:

- 1 lb. pork tenderloin.

- 3/4 teaspoon lemon pepper.

- 2 teaspoon dried oregano.

- 1 tablespoon olive oil.

- 3 tablespoon feta cheese, crumbled.

- 3 tablespoon olive tapenade.

DIRECTIONS:

1. Add pork, oil, lemon pepper, and oregano in a zip-lock bag and rub well and place in a refrigerator for 2 hours.

2. Remove pork from zip-lock bag. Using a sharp knife, make a lengthwise cut through the center of the tenderloin.

3. Spread olive tapenade on half tenderloin and sprinkle with feta cheese.

4. Fold another half of the meat over to the original shape of the tenderloin.

5. Tie close pork tenderloin with twine at 2-inch intervals.

6. Grill pork tenderloin for 20 minutes.

7. Cut into slices and serve.

NUTRITION:

- Calories: 215.

- Fat: 9.1 g.

- Carbohydrates: 1 g.

- Sugar: 0.5 g.

- Protein: 30.8 g.

- Cholesterol: 89 mg.

- **Tomatillo and Green Chili Pork Stew**

Preparation Time: 15 Minutes.

Cooking Time: 20 Minutes.

Servings: 6.

INGREDIENTS:

- 2 scallions, chopped.

- 2 cloves of garlic.

- 1 lb. tomatillos, trimmed and chopped.

- 8 large romaine or green lettuce leaves, divided.

- 2 serrano chilies, seeds, and membranes.

- ½ tsp. of dried Mexican oregano.

- 1 ½ lb. of boneless pork loin, to be cut into bite-sized cubes.

- ¼ cup of cilantro, chopped.

- ¼ tablespoon (each) salt and paper.

- 1 jalapeno, seeds and membranes to be removed and thinly sliced.

- 1 cup of sliced radishes.

- 4 lime wedges.

DIRECTIONS:

1. Combine scallions, garlic, tomatillos, 4 lettuce leaves, serrano chilies, and oregano in a blender.

2. Then puree until smooth 1-inch of puree should cover the pork; if not, add water until it covers it.

3. Season with pepper and salt, and cover it to simmer.

4. Simmer on heat for approximately 20 minutes.

NUTRITION:

- Calories: 37

- Protein: 36 g.

- Carbohydrate: 14 g.

- Fat: 19 g.

- **Plum Sauce Glazed Pork Chops**

Preparation Time: 15 Minutes.

Cooking Time: 4 hours.

Servings: 5.

INGREDIENTS:

- 6 ounces bone-free pork chops, fat trimmed.

- ¼ tsp. of salt.

- ¼ tsp. black chili pepper.

- Chinese ¼ cup plum sauce.

- 4 Yellow Mustard Teaspoons.

DIRECTIONS:

1. Season with salt and pepper to the pork chops. Cover a big, non-stick skillet over medium-high heat with cooking spray and warm.

2. Add pork chops to the skillet, and cook until the center is no longer pink, around 3 minutes per hand.

3. Combine plum sauce and mustard into a small tub. Brown the mixture and serve on top of each pork chop.

NUTRITION:

- Calories: 440.

- Fat: 33 g.

- Carbohydrates: 6 g.

- Sugar: 3 g.

- Protein: 28 g.

- Cholesterol: 97 mg.

- **Baked Pork Meatballs in Pasta Sauce**

Preparation Time: 15 Minutes.

Cooking Time: 45 Minutes.

Servings: 5.

INGREDIENTS:

- 2 lb. ground pork.
- 1 tbsp. olive oil.
- 1 cup pork rinds, crushed.
- 2 cloves garlic, minced.
- ½ cup coconut milk.
- 2 eggs, beaten.
- ½ cup Parmesan cheese, grated.
- ½ cup asiago cheese, grated.
- Salt and black pepper to taste.
- 2 jars sugar-free marinara sauce.
- 1 cup Italian blend kinds of cheeses.
- 3 tbsp. fresh basil, chopped.

DIRECTIONS:

1. Preheat oven to 400°F.
2. Combine the coconut milk and pork rinds in a bowl.
3. Mix in the ground pork, garlic, asiago cheese, Parmesan cheese, eggs, salt, and pepper and stir.
4. Form balls of the mixture and place them in a greased baking pan.
5. Bake in the oven for 20 minutes.
6. Transfer the meatballs to a plate.
7. Pour half of the marinara sauce into the baking pan.
8. Place the meatballs back in the pan and pour in the remaining marinara sauce.
9. Sprinkle with the Italian blend cheeses and drizzle with the olive oil.
10. Cover the pan with foil and put it back in the oven.
11. Bake for 10 minutes.
12. After, remove the foil, and cook for 5 minutes.
13. Once ready, take out the pan and garnish with basil.
14. Serve on a bed of squash spaghetti.

NUTRITION:

- Calories: 590.
- Fat: 46.8 g.
- Net Carbs: 4.1 g.
- Protein: 46.2 g.

- **Grilled Pork Loin Chops with Barbecue Sauce**

- Protein 34.1 g.

Preparation Time: 15 Minutes.

Cooking Time: 15 Minutes.

Servings: 5.

INGREDIENTS:

- 4 thick-cut pork loin chops, boneless.

- ½ cup sugar-free BBQ sauce.

- 1 tsp. black pepper.

- 1 tbsp. erythritol.

- ½ tsp. ginger powder.

- 2 tsp. sweet paprika.

DIRECTIONS:

1. In a bowl, mix pepper, erythritol, ginger powder, and sweet paprika, and rub the pork on all sides with the mixture.

2. Cover the pork chops with plastic wrap and place them in the fridge to marinate for 2 hours.

3. Preheat the grill to 450°F.

4. Unwrap the meat, place on the grill grate, and cook for 2 minutes per side.

5. Reduce the heat and brush the BBQ sauce on the meat, cover, and grill for 5 minutes.

6. Open the lid, turn the meat, and brush again with barbecue sauce.

7. Continue cooking covered for 5 minutes.

8. Serve.

NUTRITION:

- Calories: 363.

- Fat: 26.6 g.

- Net Carbs: 0 g.

- **Pork Pie with Cauliflower**

Preparation Time: 15 Minutes.

Cooking Time: 1 hour, 15 Minutes.

Servings: 5.

INGREDIENTS:

- 1 egg.
- ¼ cup butter.
- 2 cups almond flour.
- ¼ tsp xanthan gum.
- ¼ cup shredded mozzarella.
- A pinch of salt Filling.
- 2 lb. ground pork.
- ⅓ cup pureed onion.
- ¾ tsp. allspice.
- 1 cup mashed cauliflower.
- 1 tbsp. ground sage.
- 2 tbsp. butter.

DIRECTIONS:

1. Preheat oven to 350°F.
2. Whisk together all the crust ingredients in a bowl.
3. Make two balls out of the mixture and refrigerate for 10 minutes.
4. Combine ½ cup water, meat, and salt, in a pot over medium heat.
5. Cook for about 15 minutes.
6. Place the meat along with the other ingredients in a bowl.
7. Mix with your hands to combine.
8. Roll out the pie crusts and place one at the bottom of a greased pie pan.
9. Spread the filling over the crust.
10. Top with the other coat.
11. Bake in the oven for 50 minutes.
12. Serve.

NUTRITION:

- Calories: 325.
- Fat: 23.4 g.
- Carbohydrates: 10 g.
- Sugar: 6 g.
- Protein: 20 g.
- Cholesterol: 70 mg.

- **Pork Sausage Bake**

Preparation Time: 15 Minutes.

Cooking Time: 50 Minutes.

Servings: 4.

INGREDIENTS:

- 1 lb. pork sausages.
- 4 large tomatoes, cut in rings.
- 1 red bell pepper, sliced.
- 1 yellow bell pepper, sliced.
- 1 green bell pepper, sliced.
- 1 sprig thyme, chopped.
- 1 sprig rosemary, chopped.
- 2 cloves garlic, minced.
- 2 bay leaves.
- 2 tbsp. olive oil.
- 2 tbsp. balsamic vinegar.

DIRECTIONS:

1. Preheat oven to 350°F.
2. In a greased baking pan, arrange the tomatoes and bell peppers.
3. Sprinkle with thyme, rosemary, garlic, olive oil, and balsamic vinegar.
4. Top with the sausages.
5. Put the pan in the oven and bake for 20 minutes.
6. After, remove the pan, shake it a bit, and turn the sausages over with a spoon.
7. Continue cooking for 25 minutes or until the sausages have browned to your desired color.
8. Serve with the veggie and cooking sauce with cauli rice.

NUTRITION:

- Calories: 440.
- Fat: 33 g.
- Carbohydrates: 6 g.
- Sugar: 3 g.
- Protein: 28 g.
- Cholesterol: 97 mg.

- **Pork Osso Bucco**

Preparation Time: 15 Minutes.

Cooking Time: 1 hour, 55 Minutes.

Servings: 5.

INGREDIENTS:

- 3 tbsp. butter, softened
- 6 (16 oz.) pork shanks.
- 2 tbsp. olive oil.
- 2 cloves garlic, minced.
- 1 cup diced tomatoes.
- Salt and black pepper to taste.
- 1 onion, chopped.
- ½ celery stalk, chopped.
- ½ cup chopped carrots.
- 1 cups Cabernet Sauvignon wine.
- 3 cups vegetable broth.
- 2 tsp. lemon zest.

DIRECTIONS:

1. Melt the butter in a large saucepan over medium heat.
2. Season the pork with salt and black pepper and brown it for 12 minutes; remove to a plate.
3. In the same pan, sauté the onion for 3 minutes.
4. Return the pork shanks.
5. Stir in the wine, carrots, celery, tomatoes, broth, salt, and pepper, and cover the pan.
6. Let simmer on low heat for 1 ½ hour, basting the pork every 15 minutes with the sauce.
7. In a bowl, mix the garlic, parsley, and lemon zest to make a gremolata, and stir the mixture into the sauce when it is ready.
8. Turn the heat off and dish the Osso Bucco.
9. Serve with creamy turnip mash.

NUTRITION:

- Calories: 325. - Fat: 23.4 g.
- Carbohydrates: 10 g. - Sugar: 6 g.
- Protein: 20 g.
- Cholesterol: 70 mg.

- **Charred Tenderloin with Lemon Chimichurri**

Preparation Time: 15 Minutes.

Cooking Time: 1 hour, 15 Minutes.

Servings: 5.

INGREDIENTS:

- Lemon Chimichurri.
- 1 lemon, juiced.
- ¼ cup mint leaves, chopped.
- ¼ cup fresh oregano, chopped.
- 2 cloves garlic, minced.
- ¼ cup olive oil.
- Salt to taste.

Pork:

- 1 (4 lb.) pork tenderloin.
- Salt and black pepper to taste.
- 1 tbsp. olive oil.

DIRECTIONS:

1. Make the lemon chimichurri to have the flavors incorporate while the pork cooks.

2. In a bowl, mix the mint, oregano, and garlic.

3. Then, add the lemon juice, olive oil, and salt, and combine well. Set aside.

4. Preheat the charcoal grill to 450°F, creating a direct heat area and indirect heat area.

5. Rub the pork with olive oil and season with salt and pepper.

6. Place the meat over direct heat and sear for 3 minutes on each side, moving to the indirect heat area.

7. Close the lid and cook for 25 minutes on one side.

8. Next, open, turn the meat, and grill for 20 minutes on the other side.

9. Remove the pork from the grill and let it sit for 5 minutes before slicing.

10. Spoon lemon chimichurri over the pork and serve with fresh salad.

NUTRITION:

- Calories: 388.
- Fat: 18 g.
- Net Carbs: 2.1 g.
- Protein: 28 g.

- **Spiced Pork Roast with Collard Greens**

Preparation Time: 15 Minutes.

Cooking Time: 60 Minutes.

Servings: 5.

INGREDIENTS:

- 2 tbsp. olive oil.
- Salt and black pepper to taste.
- 1 ½ lb. pork loin.
- A pinch of dry mustard.
- 1 tsp. red pepper flakes.
- ½ tsp. ginger, minced.
- 1 cup collard greens, chopped.
- 2 garlic cloves, minced.
- ½ lemon, sliced.

DIRECTIONS:

1. In a bowl, combine the ginger with mustard, salt, and pepper.
2. Add in the meat and toss to coat.
3. Heat the oil in a saucepan over medium heat.
4. Brown the pork on all sides, about 5 minutes.
5. Transfer to the oven.
6. Pour in ¼ cup water and roast for 40 minutes at 390ºF.
7. To the saucepan, add collard greens, lemon slices, garlic, and ¼ cup water.
8. Simmer for 10 minutes.
9. Slice the loin and top with the sauce to serve.

NUTRITION:

- Calories: 440.
- Fat: 33 g.
- Carbohydrates: 6 g.
- Sugar: 3 g.
- Protein: 28 g.
- Cholesterol: 97 mg.

- **BBQ Pork Pizza with Goat Cheese**

Preparation Time: 15 Minutes.

Cooking Time: 30 Minutes.

Servings: 5.

INGREDIENTS:

- 1 low-carb pizza bread.

- 1 tbsp. olive oil.

- 1 cup Manchego cheese, grated.

- 2 cups leftover pulled pork.

- ½ cup sugar-free BBQ sauce.

- 1 cup goat cheese, crumbled.

DIRECTIONS:

1. Preheat oven to 400°F.

2. Put the pizza bread on a pizza pan.

3. Brush with olive oil and sprinkle the Manchego cheese all over.

4. Mix the pork with BBQ sauce and spread over the cheese.

5. Drop goat cheese on top and bake for 25 minutes until the cheese has melted.

6. Slice the pizza with a cutter and serve.

NUTRITION:

- Calories: 325.

- Fat: 23.4 g.

- Carbohydrates: 10 g.

- Sugar: 6 g.

- Protein: 20 g.

- Cholesterol: 70 mg.

- **Oregano Pork Chops with Spicy Tomato Sauce**

Preparation Time: 15 Minutes.

Cooking Time: 50 Minutes.

Servings: 4.

INGREDIENTS:

- 4 pork chops.
- 1 tbsp. fresh oregano, chopped.
- 2 garlic cloves, minced.
- 2 tbsp. canola oil.
- 15 oz. canned diced tomatoes.
- 1 tbsp. tomato paste.
- Salt and black pepper to taste.
- ¼ cup tomato juice.
- 1 red chili, finely chopped.

DIRECTIONS:

1. Warm the olive oil in a pan over medium heat.
2. Season the pork with salt and pepper.
3. Add it to the pan and cook for 6 minutes on both sides; remove to a bowl.
4. Sauté the garlic in the same fat for 30 seconds.
5. Stir in tomato paste, tomatoes, tomato juice, and chili.
6. Bring to a boil and reduce the heat.
7. Place in the pork chops and simmer everything for 30 minutes.
8. Sprinkle with fresh oregano and serve.

NUTRITION:

- Calories: 485.
- Fat: 41g g.
- Net Carbs: 4 g.
- Protein: 29 g.

- **Peanut Butter Pork Stir-Fry**

Preparation Time: 15 Minutes.

Cooking Time: 25 Minutes.

Servings: 4.

INGREDIENTS:

- 2 tbsp. ghee.
- 2 lb. pork loin, cut into strips.
- Pink salt to taste.
- 2 tsp. ginger-garlic paste.
- ¼ cup chicken broth.
- 5 tbsp. peanut butter, softened.
- 2 cups mixed stir-fry vegetables.
- ½ tsp. chili pepper.

DIRECTIONS:

1. Melt the ghee in a wok over high heat.
2. Rub the pork with salt, chili pepper, and ginger-garlic paste.
3. Place it into the wok and cook for 6 minutes until no longer pink.
4. Mix peanut butter and broth until smooth.
5. Pour in the wok and stir for 6 minutes.
6. Add in the mixed veggies and simmer for 5 minutes.
7. Adjust the taste with salt and black pepper and spoon the stir-fry to a side of cilantro cauli rice.

NUTRITION:

- Calories: 440.
- Fat: 33 g.
- Carbohydrates: 6 g.
- Sugar: 3 g.
- Protein: 28 g.
- Cholesterol: 97 mg.

6. Cook for 25 minutes, at 390°F.

7. After halftime, take the basket out and spray the chicken with olive oil

8. This step is optional. Mix two tbsp. Of hot sauce with melted butter. Brush the cooked crispy chicken with it.

9. Serve with the spinach salad.

NUTRITION:

- Calories: 330.

- Fat: 20 g.

- Carbs: 19 g.

- Protein: 26 g.

POULTRY

- **Air Fryer Nashville Hot Chicken with Spinach Salad**

Preparation Time: 30 Minutes.

Cooking Time: 25 Minutes.

Servings: 8.

INGREDIENTS:

- 2 cups Buttermilk.

- 8 Chicken thighs, bone-in.

- 1 tsp. Cayenne pepper.

- 1/4 cup Hot sauce.

- 2 Tbsp. Garlic powder.

- 1 tsp. Salt.

- 1/2 cup Low-fat butter.

- 2 cups Flour.

- 1 tsp. Black pepper.

- 1 tsp. Old bay.

- 1 tsp. Paprika.

DIRECTIONS:

1. In a mixing bowl, add hot sauce and buttermilk, mix it well, then add chicken pieces.

2. Marinate in the refrigerator for 1 to 24 hours. Mix all the ingredients.

3. Take chicken out from buttermilk, coat in the flour mix.

4. Let the chicken rest on a cooling rack for 15 minutes before putting it in the air fryer.

5. Place the breaded chicken in the air fryer, leaving room between the pieces.

- **Air Fryer Italian Sausage & Vegetables**

Preparation Time: 5 Minutes.

Cooking Time: 15 Minutes.

Servings: 5.

INGREDIENTS:

- 1 bell pepper.
- 4 pieces spicy or sweet Italian Sausage.
- 1 small onion.
- 1/4 cup of mushrooms.

DIRECTIONS:

1. Let the air fryer preheat to 400°F for three minutes.
2. Put Italian sausage in a single layer in the air fryer basket and let it cook for six minutes.
3. Slice the vegetables while the sausages are cooking.
4. After six minutes, reduce the temperature to 360°F. flip the sausage halfway through. Add the mushrooms, onions, and peppers in the basket around the sausage.
5. Cook at 360°F for 8 minutes. After a 4-minute mix around the sausage and vegetables.
6. With an instant-read thermometer, the sausage temperature should be 160°F.
7. Cook more for few minutes if the temperature is not 160°F.
8. Take vegetables and sausage out and serve hot with brown rice.

NUTRITION:

- Calories: 291.
- Fat: 21 g.
- Carbs: 10 g.
- Protein: 16 g.

- **Spinach Chicken Cheesy Bake**

Preparation Time: 5 Minutes.

Cooking Time: 45 Minutes.

Servings: 3.

INGREDIENTS:

- 1 lb. chicken breasts.
- 1 tsp. mixed spice seasoning.
- Pink salt and black pepper to taste.
- 2 loose cups baby spinach.
- 3 tsp. olive oil.
- 4 oz. cream cheese.
- 1 ¼ cups mozzarella cheese, grated.
- 4 tbsp. water.

DIRECTIONS:

1. Preheat oven to 370°F.
2. Season chicken with spice mix, salt, and black pepper.
3. Pat with your hands to have the seasoning stick on the chicken.
4. Put in the casserole dish and layer spinach over the chicken.
5. Mix the oil with cream cheese, mozzarella, salt, and pepper and stir in water a tablespoon at a time.
6. Pour the mixture over the chicken and cover the casserole dish with aluminum foil. Bake for 20 minutes.
7. Remove the foil and continue cooking for 15 minutes until a nice golden brown color is formed on top.
8. Take out and allow sitting for 5 minutes.
9. Serve warm with braised asparagus.

NUTRITION:

- Calories: 233.
- Fat: 7 g.
- Carbs: 26 g.
- Protein: 18 g.

- **Air Fryer Chicken Wings with Buffalo Sauce**

Preparation Time: 5 Minutes.

Cooking Time: 30 Minutes.

Servings: 5.

INGREDIENTS:

- 4 cups Chicken drumettes and flats.
- Salt & pepper, to taste.

Buffalo Sauce:

- 1/2 cup hot sauce.
- 2 tablespoons White vinegar.
- 1/2 cup Melted butter.
- 2 teaspoons Worcestershire sauce.
- Pinch of garlic powder.

DIRECTIONS:

1. Let the air fryer preheat to 380°F.
2. Separate the wings, making a flat and drumsticks, discarding the tips.
3. With paper towels, pat dry the chicken wings, sprinkle generously salt and pepper, and other seasonings of your choice.
4. Put them in an air-fryer basket and cook for about 22 minutes.
5. After that increase, the temperature to 400°F, cook for five more minutes for chicken skin to get crispy.
6. Mix all ingredients of buffalo sauce and mix well.
7. Coat the wings with homemade buffalo sauce.
8. Serve with the side of salad greens.

NUTRITION:

- Calories: 315.
- Fat: 20 g.
- Carbs: 1 g.
- Protein: 30 g.

- **Air Fryer Grilled Chicken Recipe**

Preparation Time: 20 Minutes.

Cooking Time: 30 Minutes.

Servings: 4.

INGREDIENTS:

- 4 cups Chicken tenders.
- Marinade.
- 2 tbsp. Honey.
- 1/4 cup Olive oil.
- 2 tbsp. White vinegar.
- 2 tbsp. Water.
- ½ tsp. salt.
- 1 tsp. Garlic powder.
- Half teaspoon of paprika.
- 1 tsp. Onion powder.
- ½ tsp. crushed red pepper.

DIRECTIONS:

1. In a mixing bowl, add all ingredients of the marinade and mix well.
2. Then add the chicken mix to coat. Cover with plastic wrap, and marinate in the refrigerator for half an hour.
3. Put chicken tenders in the air fryer basket in one even layer.
4. Cook for 3 minutes at 390°F. flip the tenders over and cook for five minutes more or until the chicken is completely cooked through.
5. Serve with the side of salad greens.

NUTRITION:

- Calories: 230.
- Fat: 14 g.
- Protein: 20 g.
- Carbs: 11 g.

- **Air-Fried Chicken Pie**

Preparation Time: 5 Minutes.

Cooking Time: 30 Minutes.

Servings: 2.

INGREDIENTS:

- 2 sheets puff pastry.
- 2 pieces chicken thighs, cut into cubes.
- 1 small onion, chopped.
- 2 small potatoes, chopped.
- 1/4 cup Mushrooms.
- Light soya sauce.
- 1 carrot.
- Black pepper, to taste.
- Worcestershire sauce, to taste.
- Salt, to taste.
- Italian mixed dried herbs.
- A pinch garlic powder.
- 2 tbsp. plain flour.
- Milk, as required.
- Melted butter.

DIRECTIONS:

1. In a mixing bowl, add light soya sauce and pepper, add the chicken cubes, and coat well.

2. In a pan over medium heat, sauté carrot, potatoes, and onion. Add some water, if required, to cook the vegetables.

3. Add the chicken cubes and mushrooms and cook them too.

4. Stir in black pepper, salt, Worcestershire sauce, garlic powder, and dried herbs.

5. When the chicken is cooked through, add some of the flour and mix well.

6. Add in the milk and let the vegetables simmer until tender.

7. Place one piece of puff pastry in the baking tray of the air fryer, poke holes with a fork.

8. Add on top the cooked chicken filling and eggs and puff pastry on top, with holes. Cut the excess pastry off. Glaze with oil spray or melted butter

9. Air fry at 180°F for six minutes or until it becomes golden brown.

10. Serve with microgreens.

NUTRITION:

- Calories: 224.
- Protein: 20 g.
- Fat: 18 g.
- Carbs: 17 g.

- **Air-Fried Buttermilk Chicken**

Preparation Time: 20 Minutes.

Cooking Time: 30 Minutes.

Servings: 5.

INGREDIENTS:

- 4 cups skin-on, bone-in Chicken thighs.

Marinade:

- 2 cups Buttermilk.
- 2 tsp. Black pepper.
- 1 tsp. Cayenne pepper.
- 2 tsp. Salt.

Seasoned Flour:

- 1 tbsp. Baking powder.
- 2 cups All-purpose flour.
- 1 tbsp. Paprika powder.
- 1 tsp. Salt.
- 1 tbsp. Garlic powder.

DIRECTIONS:

1. Let the air fry heat at 180°C.
2. With a paper towel, pat dry the chicken thighs.
3. In a mixing bowl, add paprika, black pepper, salt mix well, then add chicken pieces. Add buttermilk and coat the chicken well. Let it marinate for at least 6 hours.
4. In another bowl, add baking powder, salt, flour, pepper, and paprika. Put one by one of the chicken pieces and coat in the seasoning mix.
5. Spray oil on chicken pieces and place breaded chicken skin side up in air fryer basket in one layer, cook for 8 minutes, then flip the chicken pieces' cook for another ten minutes
6. Take out and serve with salad greens.

NUTRITION:

- Calories: 210.
- Fat: 18 g.
- Protein: 22 g.
- Carbs: 12 g.

- **Low Carb Parmesan Chicken Meatballs**

- Carbs: 12.1 g.
- Protein: 19.9 g.

Preparation Time: 15 Minutes.

Cooking Time: 15 Minutes.

Servings: 20.

INGREDIENTS:

- Half cup, ground pork rinds.
- 4 cups ground chicken.
- ½ cup grated parmesan cheese.
- 1 tsp. kosher salt.
- 1 tsp. garlic powder.
- 1 egg beaten
- 1 tsp. paprika.
- ½ tsp. pepper.

Breading:

- Pork rinds: ½ cup ground.

DIRECTIONS:

1. Let the Air Fryer preheat to 400°F.
2. Add cheese, chicken, egg, pepper, and ½ cup of pork rinds, garlic, salt, and paprika in a big mixing ball. Mix well into a dough, make into 1and half-inch balls.
3. Coat the meatballs in pork rinds (ground).
4. Oil sprays the air fry basket and add meatballs in one even layer.
5. Let it cook for 12 minutes at 400°F, flipping once halfway through.
6. Serve with salad greens.

NUTRITION:

- Calories: 240.
- Fat: 10 g.

- **Sriracha-Honey Chicken Wings**

Preparation Time: 10 Minutes.

Cooking Time: 15 Minutes.

Servings: 4.

INGREDIENTS:

- 1 and 1/2 tablespoons soy sauce.
- 4 cups chicken wings.
- 2 tablespoons sriracha sauce.
- 1 tablespoon butter.
- ½ cup honey.
- Juice of half lime.
- Scallion's cilantro, and chives for garnish.

DIRECTIONS:

1. Let the air fryer preheat to 360°F.
2. Put the chicken wings into an air fryer basket, cook for half an hour, flip the wings every seven minutes, and cook thoroughly.
3. Meanwhile, in a saucepan, add all the ingredients of the sauce and simmer for three minutes.
4. Take out the chicken wings and coat them in sauce well.
5. Garnish with scallions. Serve with a microgreen salad.

NUTRITION:

- Calories: 207.
- Proteins: 22 g.
- Carbs: 10 g.
- Fat: 15 g.

- **Air Fryer Chicken Cheese Quesadilla**

Preparation Time: 5 Minutes.

Cooking Time: 7 Minutes.

Servings: 5.

INGREDIENTS:

- 1 cup, diced pre-cooked chicken.
- 2 pieces tortillas.
- 1 cup (shredded) low-fat cheese.

DIRECTIONS:

1. Spray oil into the air basket and place one tortilla in it. Add cooked chicken and cheese on top.
2. Add the second tortilla on top. Put a metal rack on top.
3. Cook for 6 minutes at 370°F, flip it halfway through so cooking evenly.
4. Slice and serve with salad greens.

NUTRITION:

- Calories: 171.
- Carbohydrates: 8 g.
- Protein: 15 g.
- Fat: 8 g.

- **Air Fried Empanadas**

Preparation Time: 5 Minutes.

Cooking Time: 20 Minutes.

Servings: 2.

INGREDIENTS

- 8 pieces square gyoza wrappers.
- 1 tablespoon olive oil.
- 1/4 cup, finely diced white onion.
- 1/4 cup, finely diced mushrooms.
- 1/2 cup lean ground beef.
- 2 teaspoons chopped garlic.
- 1/4 teaspoon paprika.
- 1/4 teaspoon ground cumin.
- 6 green olives, diced.
- 1/8 teaspoon ground cinnamon.
- 1/2 cup diced tomatoes.
- 1 egg, lightly beaten.

DIRECTIONS:

1. In a skillet, over a medium flame, add oil, onions, and beef and cook for 3 minutes, until beef turns brown.

2. Add mushrooms, and cook for six minutes until it starts to brown. Then add paprika, cinnamon, olives, cumin, and garlic and cook for 3 minutes or more.

3. Add in the chopped tomatoes, and cook for a minute. Turn off the heat; let it cool for five minutes.

4. Lay gyoza wrappers on a flat surface add one and a half tbsp. of beef filling in each wrapper. Brush edges with water or egg, fold wrappers, pinch edges.

5. Put four empanadas in an even layer in an air fryer basket, and cook for 7 minutes at 400°F until nicely browned.

6. Serve with sauce and salad greens.

NUTRITION:

- Calories: 343.
- Fat: 19 g.
- Protein: 18 g.
- Carbohydrates: 12.9 g.

- **Air Fryer BBQ Chicken Wings**

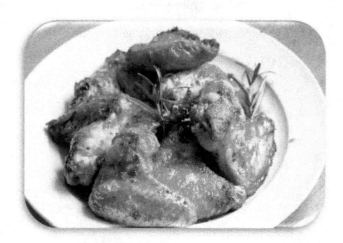

Preparation Time: 5 Minutes.

Cooking Time: 15 Minutes.

Servings: 4.

INGREDIENTS:

- BBQ sauce: half cup.
- Chicken wings: 4 cups.
- Black pepper, to taste.
- Garlic powder: 1/8 teaspoon.
- Ranch.
- Celery sticks.

DIRECTIONS:

1. Let Air Fryer preheat to 400°F.

2. With paper towels, pat dry the chicken wings, rub the garlic powder on them. Put them in the air fryer, in one even layer.

3. Let it cook for 15 minutes; flip the wings once or twice. Cook for another 3 minutes for crispy skin.

4. Take them out from the air fryer and toss them in BBQ sauce. Toss well to coat.

5. Serve with celery sticks, mixed greens, and ranch dressing.

NUTRITION:

- Calories: 197.
- Carbohydrates: 14 g.
- Protein: 11 g.
- Fat: 10 g.

- **Air Fryer Cornish Hen**

Preparation Time: 5 Minutes.

Cooking Time: 25 Minutes.

Servings: 5.

INGREDIENTS:

- One Cornish hen
- Salt & black pepper, to taste
- Olive oil spray
- Paprika, ¼ tbsp.

DIRECTIONS:

1. Mix all spices and Rub the spices all over Cornish hen.
2. Spray the air fryer basket with olive oil.
3. Put Cornish hen in an Air fryer.
4. Cook for 25 minutes at 390° F. flip after half time.
5. Serve with a mixed green salad.

NUTRITION:

- Calories: 300.
- Protein: 25 g.
- Fat: 21 g.
- Carbs: 20 g.

- **Ghee Chicken Mix**

Preparation Time: 10 Minutes.

Cooking Time: 20 Minutes.

Servings: 4.

INGREDIENTS:

- 2 tablespoons garlic powder.

- 2 chicken breasts, skinless boneless and sliced.

- Salt and black pepper to the taste.

- ½ cup ghee, melted.

- ½ cup chicken stock.

- 1 tablespoon cilantro.

DIRECTIONS:

1. Heat up a pan with the ghee over medium heat, add the chicken and cook for 5 minutes on each side.

2. Add the rest of the ingredients, cook for 10 minutes more, divide between plates and serve.

NUTRITION:

- Calories: 439.

- Fat: 33.4 g.

- Fiber: 0.4 g.

- Carbs: 3.2 g.

- Protein: 31.3 g.

- **Paprika Chicken Wings**

Preparation Time: 10 Minutes.

Cooking Time: 20 Minutes.

Servings: 5.

INGREDIENTS:

- 1 pound chicken wings.
- 1 tablespoon cumin, ground.
- 1 teaspoon coriander, ground.
- 1 tablespoon sweet paprika.
- A pinch of salt and black pepper.
- 1 tablespoon lime juice.
- 2 tablespoons olive oil.

DIRECTIONS:

1. In a bowl, mix the chicken wings with the cumin and the other ingredients, toss, and spread them on a baking sheet lined with parchment paper and cook at 420°F for 20 minutes.
2. Divide between plates and serve.

NUTRITION:

- Calories: 286.
- Fat: 16 g.
- Fiber: 0.8 g.
- Carbs: 1.6 g.
- Protein: 33.3 g.

- **Chicken and Capers**

Preparation Time: 10 Minutes.

Cooking Time: 15 Minutes.

Servings: 5.

INGREDIENTS

- 1 pound chicken breast, skinless, boneless, and sliced.
- 1 tablespoon olive oil.
- 1 tablespoons capers, drained.
- 1 cup tomato passata.
- A pinch of salt and black pepper.
- 1 tablespoon parsley, chopped.

DIRECTIONS:

1. Heat up a pan on medium heat, add the chicken and cook for 4 minutes on each side.
2. Add the rest of the ingredients, cook for 8 minutes more, divide between plates and serve.

NUTRITION:

- Calories: 166.
- Fat: 6.4 g.
- Fiber: 0.6 g.
- Carbs: 1.2 g.
- Protein: 24.6 g.

- **Cilantro Wings**

Preparation Time: 10 Minutes.

Cooking Time: 25 Minutes.

Servings: 5.

INGREDIENTS:

- 2 pounds chicken wings.

- Juice of 1 lime.

- 1 tablespoon olive oil.

- ¼ cup cilantro, chopped.

- 2 garlic cloves, minced.

- A pinch of salt and black pepper.

DIRECTIONS:

1. In a bowl, mix the chicken wings with the lime juice and the other ingredients, toss and transfer them to a roasting pan.

2. Introduce in the oven and cook at 390° F for 20 minutes.

3. Divide the chicken wings between plates and serve with a side dish.

NUTRITION:

- Calories: 463.

- Fat: 20.3 g.

- Fiber: 0.1 g.

- Carbs: 0.6 g.

- Protein: 65.7 g.

- **Baked Turkey Mix**

Preparation Time: 10 Minutes.

Cooking Time: 30 Minutes.

Servings: 4.

INGREDIENTS:

- 1 big turkey breast, skinless, boneless, and sliced.
- 3 green onions, chopped.
- ½ cup tomato passata.
- 1 tablespoon avocado oil.
- 1 cup green olives, pitted and halved.
- 2 tablespoons parmesan, grated.

DIRECTIONS:

1. Grease a baking dish with the oil, arrange the turkey slices inside, add the onions and the other ingredients except for the parmesan, and toss.
2. Sprinkle the parmesan on top, introduce the dish to the oven and bake at 390°F for 30 minutes.
3. Divide the mix between plates and serve.

NUTRITION:

- Calories: 450 g.
- Fat: 24 g.
- Fiber: 0 g.
- Carbs: 3 g.
- Protein: 60 g.

- **Turkey and Artichokes Mix**

Preparation Time: 10 Minutes.

Cooking Time: 25 Minutes.

Servings: 5.

INGREDIENTS:

- 2 tablespoons olive oil.
- 1 red onion, chopped.
- 1 cup chicken stock.
- 1 big turkey breast, skinless, boneless, and sliced.
- 2 artichokes, trimmed and quartered.
- 4 garlic cloves, minced.
- A pinch of salt and black pepper.
- ½ teaspoon red chili flakes.
- 1 tablespoon cilantro.

DIRECTIONS:

1. Heat up a pan with the oil, add the turkey and cook for 5 minutes.
2. Add the onion and the other ingredients, cook everything over medium heat for 20 minutes more, divide between plates and serve.

NUTRITION

- Calories: 400.
- Fat: 20 g.
- Fiber: 1 g.
- Carbs: 2 g.
- Protein: 7 g.

- **Curry Chicken**

Preparation Time: 10 Minutes.

Cooking Time: 30 Minutes.

Servings: 5.

INGREDIENTS:

- 1 pound chicken breast, skinless, boneless, and cubed.
- 1 tablespoon olive oil.
- 1 tablespoon yellow curry paste.
- 1 cup chicken stock.
- A pinch of salt and black pepper.
- 1 teaspoon sweet paprika.
- ½ teaspoon allspice, ground.
- 1 tablespoon cilantro, chopped.

DIRECTIONS:

1. Heat up a pan, add the meat and brown it for 5 minutes.
2. Add the curry paste and the other ingredients, toss, bring to a simmer and cook for 25 minutes.
3. Divide the mix into bowls and serve.

NUTRITION:

- Calories: 334.
- Fat: 24 g.
- Fiber: 2 g.
- Carbs: 4.5 g.
- Protein: 27 g.

- **Turkey and Coconut Sauce**

Preparation Time: 10 Minutes.

Cooking Time: 30 Minutes.

Servings: 4.

INGREDIENTS:

- 1 tablespoon coconut oil, melted.
- 1 turkey breast, skinless, boneless, and cubed.
- 1 cup chicken stock.
- 2 shallots, chopped.
- ¼ cup coconut milk.
- 2 tablespoons parsley, chopped.
- A pinch of salt and black pepper.

DIRECTIONS:

1. Heat up a pan with the oil over medium-high heat, add the shallots and the meat, and brown for 5 minutes.
2. Add the stock and the other ingredients, bring to a simmer, and cook for 25 minutes, stirring often.
3. Divide into bowls and serve.

NUTRITION:

- Calories: 112.
- Fat: 7.9 g.
- Fiber: 0.6 g.
- Carbs: 3 g.
- Protein: 7.9 g.

- **Coriander Chicken Mix**

Preparation Time: 10 Minutes.

Cooking Time: 20 Minutes.

Servings: 4.

INGREDIENTS:

- 2 pounds chicken breasts, skinless, boneless, and cubed.
- 2 teaspoons cumin, ground.
- 2 tablespoons avocado oil.
- 2 tablespoons lime juice.
- A pinch of salt and black pepper.
- 1 teaspoon coriander, ground.
- 1 tablespoon cilantro.

DIRECTIONS:

1. Heat the pan, add the chicken and brown it for 5 minutes.
2. Add the cumin and the other ingredients, toss, cook over medium heat for 15 minutes more, divide between plates and serve with a side salad.

NUTRITION:

- Calories: 240.
- Fat: 10 g.
- Fiber: 2 g.
- Carbs: 5 g.
- Protein: 20 g.

- **Baked Tarragon Turkey**

Preparation Time: 10 Minutes.

Cooking Time: 30 Minutes.

Servings: 4.

INGREDIENTS:

- 1 pound turkey breast.
- 2 tablespoons olive oil.
- 1 cup chicken stock.
- A pinch of salt and black pepper.
- 1 tablespoon tarragon, chopped.

DIRECTIONS:

1. In a roasting pan, combine the meat with the oil and the other ingredients,
2. Bake at 390°F for 30 minutes.
3. Divide the turkey mix between plates and serve with a side salad.

NUTRITION:

- Calories: 182.
- Fat: 9.1 g.
- Fiber: 0.6 g.
- Carbs: 5.2 g.
- Protein: 19.6 g.

- **Chicken and Salsa**

Preparation Time: 10 Minutes.

Cooking Time: 20 Minutes.

Servings: 4.

INGREDIENTS:

- 2 pounds chicken breasts, skinless, boneless, and cubed.
- 2 tablespoons olive oil.
- ½ cup chicken stock.
- 2 shallots, chopped.
- 1 cup cherry tomatoes, halved.
- 1 cup cucumber, cubed.
- 1 cup black olives, pitted and sliced.
- ¼ cup parsley, chopped.
- 1 tablespoon lime juice.

DIRECTIONS:

1. Heat up a pan, add the shallots, toss and cook for 2 minutes.
2. Add the chicken and brown for 5 minutes more.
3. Add the tomatoes and the other ingredients, toss, cook over medium heat for 12–13 minutes more, divide into bowls and serve.

NUTRITION:

- Calories: 230.
- Fat: 12 g.
- Fiber: 5.0 g.
- Carbs: 6.3 g.
- Protein: 20 g.

- **Creamy Turkey**

Preparation Time: 10 Minutes.

Cooking Time: 30 Minutes.

Servings: 5.

INGREDIENTS:

- 1 pound turkey breast.

- 1 cup heavy cream.

- 2 tablespoons olive oil.

- 2 spring onions, chopped.

- 2 leeks, chopped.

- A pinch of salt and black pepper.

- 1 tablespoon cilantro.

DIRECTIONS:

1. Heat up a pan with the oil, add the spring onions and the leeks and sauté for 2 minutes.

2. Add the meat and brown for 3 minutes more.

3. Add the rest of the ingredients, bring to a simmer and cook over medium heat for 25 minutes more, stirring often.

4. Divide the mix into bowls and serve.

NUTRITION:

- Calories: 267.

- Fat: 5.6 g.

- Fiber: 0 g.

- Carbs: 6.0 g.

- Protein: 35 g.

SEAFOOD

- **Baked Fish Fillets**

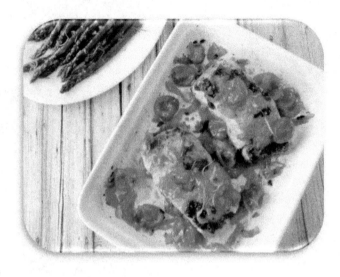

Preparation Time: 5 Minutes.

Cooking Time: 20 Minutes.

Servings: 2.

INGREDIENTS:

- 2 tablespoons butter, melted.
- A pinch ground paprika.
- 3 fish fillets (5 ounces).
- Pepper to taste.
- 1 tablespoon lemon juice.
- ½ teaspoon salt.

DIRECTIONS:

1. Make sure that your oven is preheated to 350°F.
2. Prepare a baking pan by greasing it with some fat.
3. Sprinkle salt and pepper over the fillets and place them in the pan.
4. Add butter, paprika, and lemon juice into a bowl and stir. Brush this mixture over the fillets.
5. Place the baking pan in the oven and bake the fillets for 15–25 minutes, until the fish flakes easily when pierced with a fork.

NUTRITION:

- Calories: 245.
- Fat: 12 g.
- Carbs: 4 g.
- Protein: 32 g.
- Sodium: 455 g.

- **Salmon Cakes**

Preparation Time: 10 Minutes.

Cooking Time: 10 Minutes.

Servings: 2.

INGREDIENTS:

- 2 cans salmon (14.75 ounces each), drained.
- 8 tablespoons collagen.
- 2 cups shredded mozzarella cheese.
- 1 teaspoon onion powder.
- 4 large pastured eggs.
- 4 teaspoons dried dill.
- 1 teaspoon pink sea salt or to taste.
- 4 tablespoons bacon grease.

DIRECTIONS:

1. Add salmon, collagen, mozzarella, onion powder, eggs, dill, and salt into a bowl and mix well.
2. Make 8 patties from the mixture.
3. Place a large skillet over a medium-low flame with bacon grease. Once the fat is well heated, place the salmon cakes in the skillet and cook until it becomes golden brown on all sides.
4. Take off the pan from heat and let the patties remain in the cooked fat for 5 minutes. Serve.

NUTRITION:

- Calories: 245.
- Fat: 12 g.
- Carbs: 4 g.
- Protein: 32 g.
- Sodium: 455 g.

- **Fish Bone Broth**

Preparation Time: 10 Minutes.

Cooking Time: 10 minutes.

Servings: 2.

INGREDIENTS:

- 2 pounds of fish head or carcass.
- Salt to taste.
- 7–8 quarts water + extra to blanch.
- 2 inches ginger, sliced.
- 2 tablespoons lemon juice.

DIRECTIONS:

1. To blanch the fish: Add water and fish heads into a large pot. Place the pot over high heat.
2. When it boils, turn the heat off and discard the water.
3. Place the fish back in the pot. Pour 7–8 quarts of water.
4. Place the pot over high heat. Add ginger, salt, and lemon juice.
5. When the mixture boils, reduce the heat and cover with a lid. Simmer for 4 hours.
6. Remove from heat. When it cools down, strain into a large jar with a wire mesh strainer.
7. Refrigerate for 5–6 days. Unused broth can be frozen.

NUTRITION:

- Calories: 207 g.
- Proteins: 22g g.
- Carbs: 10g g.
- Fat: 15 g.

- **Garlic Butter Shrimp**

Preparation Time: 10 Minutes.

Cooking Time: 10 Minutes.

Servings: 2.

INGREDIENTS:

- 1 cup unsalted butter, divided.

- Kosher salt to taste.

- ½ cup chicken stock.

- Freshly ground pepper to taste.

- ¼ cup chopped fresh parsley leaves.

- 3 pounds medium shrimp, peeled, deveined.

- Garlic.

- Juice of 2 lemons.

DIRECTIONS:

1. Add 4 tablespoons butter into a large skillet and place the skillet over medium-high flame. Once butter melts, stir in salt, shrimp, and pepper and cook for 2–3 minutes. Stir every minute or so. Remove shrimp with a slotted spoon and place on a plate.

2. Add garlic into the pot and cook until you get a nice aroma. Pour lemon juice and stock and stir.

3. Once it comes to a boil, lower the heat and cook until the stock reduces to half its initial quantity.

4. Add the rest of the butter, a tablespoon each time, and stir until it melts each time.

5. Add shrimp and stir lightly until well coated.

6. Sprinkle parsley on top and serve.

NUTRITION:

- Cal 233

- Fat: 7 g.

- Carbs: 26 g.

- Protein: 18 g.

- **Grilled Shrimp**

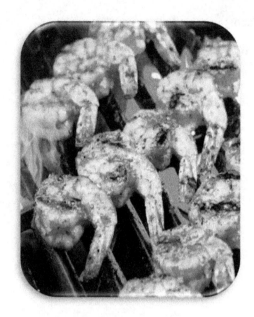

Preparation Time: 10 Minutes.

Cooking Time: 5 Minutes.

Servings: 2.

INGREDIENTS:

- 2 teaspoons garlic powder.
- 2 teaspoons Italian seasoning.
- 2 teaspoons kosher salt.
- ½ - 1 teaspoon cayenne pepper.

Grilling:

- 4 tablespoons extra-virgin olive oil.
- 2 pounds shrimp, peeled, deveined.
- 2 tablespoons fresh lemon juice.
- Oil to grease the grill grated.

DIRECTIONS:

1. You can grill the shrimp in a grill or boil it in an oven. Choose whatever method suits you and preheat the grill or oven to high heat.

2. In case you are broiling it in an oven, prepare a baking sheet by lining it with foil and greasing the foil as well, with some fat.

3. Add garlic powder, cayenne pepper, salt, and Italian seasoning into a large bowl and mix well.

4. Add lemon juice and oil and mix well.

5. Stir in the shrimp. Make sure that the shrimp are well coated with the mixture.

6. If using the grill, fix the shrimp on skewers else, place them on the baking sheet.

7. Grease the grill grates with some oil. Grill the shrimp or broil them in an oven until they turn pink. It should take 2–3 minutes for each side.

NUTRITION:

- Calories: 245.
- Fat: 12 g.
- Carbs: 4 g.
- Protein: 32 g.
- Sodium: 455 g.

- **Garlic Ghee Pan-Fried Cod**

Preparation Time: 5 Minutes.

Cooking Time: 10 Minutes.

Servings: 2.

INGREDIENTS:

- 2 cod fillets (4.8 ounces each).
- 3 cloves garlic, peeled, minced.
- Salt to taste.
- 1 ½ tablespoons ghee.
- ½ tablespoon garlic powder (optional).

DIRECTIONS:

1. Place a pan over medium-high flame. Add ghee.
2. Once ghee melts, stir in half the garlic and cook for about 6–10 seconds.
3. Add fillets and season with garlic powder and salt.
4. Soon the color of fish will turn absolutely white. This color should be visible for about half the height of the fish.
5. Turn the fish over and cook, adding remaining garlic.
6. When the entire fillet turns white, remove it from the pan, and serve.

NUTRITION:

- Calories: 207 g.
- Proteins: 22g g.
- Carbs: 10g g.
- Fat: 15 g.

- **Mussel and Potato Stew**

Preparation Time: 10 Minutes.

Cooking Time: 20 Minutes.

Servings: 5.

INGREDIENTS:

- Potatoes.

- Broccoli.

- Olive oil.

- Filets.

- Garlic.

DIRECTIONS:

1. Submerge potatoes in cold water in a medium saucepan. Put the salt, and boil. Allow to cook for 15 minutes till soft. Let drain.

2. Boil a saucepan of salted water. Put broccoli rabe, and allow to cook till just soft; it should turn bright green. Drain thoroughly, and slice into 2-inch lengths.

3. In a big, deep skillet, mix garlic, anchovies, and oil. Let cook over high heat for approximately a minute, crushing anchovies. In a skillet, scatter the mussels, put chopped parsley, broccoli rabe, and potatoes on top. Put half cup water, and add salt to season. Place the cover, and allow to cook till mussels are open. Serve.

NUTRITION:

- Calories: 233.

- Fat: 7 g.

- Carbs: 26 g.

- Protein: 18 g.

- **Tuna and Tomatoes**

Preparation Time: 5 Minutes

Cooking Time: 20 Minutes

Servings: 2

INGREDIENTS:

- 1 yellow onion, chopped.

- 1 tablespoon olive oil.

- 1 pound tuna fillets, boneless, skinless, and cubed.

- 1 cup tomatoes, chopped.

- 1 red pepper, chopped.

- 1 teaspoon sweet paprika.

- 1 tablespoon coriander, chopped.

DIRECTIONS:

1. Heat up a pan with the oil over medium heat, add the onions and the pepper and cook for 5 minutes.

2. Add the fish and the other ingredients, cook everything for 15 minutes, divide between plates and serve.

NUTRITION:

- Calories: 245.

- Fat: 12 g.

- Carbs: 4 g.

- Protein: 32 g.

- Sodium: 455 g.

- **Mustard Salmon with Herbs**

Preparation Time: 10 Minutes.

Cooking Time: 30 Minutes.

Servings: 2.

INGREDIENTS:

- Mustard.

- Mayonnaise.

- Dressing mix.

- Garlic powder, or to taste.

- Lemons.

- Salmon fillet.

- 1 sprig fresh mint, stemmed, or to taste.

- 1 sprig fresh rosemary, or to taste.

- 2 tablespoons chopped fresh chives, or to taste.

- 1 sprig fresh dill, or to taste.

- 4 cloves garlic, crushed, or to taste.

DIRECTIONS:

1. In a bowl, combine garlic powder, ranch dressing, Italian dressing, mayonnaise, and mustard. Squeeze over the mixture with 1/2 of the lemon. Cut the leftover lemon halves.

2. Put in the preheated oven and bake for 30–45 minutes until a fork can easily flake the flesh. Gently open the foil and remove the herb sprigs before eating.

NUTRITION:

- Calories: 207 g.

- Proteins: 22g g.

- Carbs: 10g g.

- Fat: 15g g.

- **Nutty Coconut Fish**

Preparation Time: 5 Minutes.

Cooking Time: 30 Minutes.

Servings: 3.

INGREDIENTS:

- Mayonnaise.

- Mustard.

- Bread crumbs.

- Shredded coconut.

- Mixed nuts.

- Granulated sugar.

- 1 teaspoon salt.

- 1/2 teaspoon cayenne pepper.

- 1 pound whitefish fillets.

DIRECTIONS

1. Preheat the oven to 190°C/375°F. Grease the medium baking dish lightly.

2. Blend brown mustard and mayonnaise in a small bowl. Mix cayenne pepper, salt, sugar, chopped mixed nuts, shredded coconut, and dry breadcrumbs in a medium bowl.

3. Dip fish in mayonnaise mixture, then dip in breadcrumb mixture. In the prepped baking dish, put coated fish fillets.

4. Bake in preheated oven for 20 minutes until fish flakes easily with a fork.

NUTRITION:

- Calories: 233.

- Fat: 7 g.

- Carbs: 26 g.

- Protein: 18 g.

- **Creamy Mackerel**

Preparation Time: 10 Minutes.

Cooking Time: 20 Minutes.

Servings: 4.

INGREDIENTS:

- 2 shallots, minced.

- 2 spring onions, chopped.

- 2 tablespoons olive oil.

- 4 mackerel fillets, skinless and cut into medium cubes.

- 1 cup heavy cream.

- 1 teaspoon cumin, ground.

- ½ teaspoon oregano, dried.

- A pinch of salt and black pepper.

- 2 tablespoons chives, chopped.

DIRECTIONS:

1. Heat up a pan with the oil over medium heat, add the spring onions and the shallots, stir and sauté for 5 minutes.

2. Add the fish and cook it for 4 minutes.

3. Add the rest of the ingredients, bring to a simmer, cook everything for 10 minutes more, divide between plates, and serve.

NUTRITION:

- Calories: 403 g.

- Fat: 33.9 g.

- Fiber: 0.4 g.

- Carbs: 2.7 g.

- Protein: 22 g.

- **Turmeric Tilapia**

Preparation Time: 10 Minutes.

Cooking Time: 15 Minutes.

Servings: 5.

INGREDIENTS:

- 4 tilapia fillets, boneless.

- 2 tablespoons olive oil.

- 1 teaspoon turmeric powder.

- A pinch of salt and black pepper.

- 2 spring onions, chopped.

- ¼ teaspoon basil, dried.

- ¼ teaspoon garlic powder.

- 1 tablespoon parsley, chopped.

DIRECTIONS:

1. Heat up a pan with the oil over medium heat, add the spring onions and cook them for 2 minutes.

2. Add the fish, turmeric, and the other ingredients, cook for 5 minutes on each side, divide between plates and serve.

NUTRITION:

- Calories: 205.

- Fat: 8.6 g.

- Fiber: 0.4 g.

- Carbs: 1.1 g.

- Protein: 31.8 g.

- **Walnut Salmon Mix**

Preparation Time: 10 Minutes.

Cooking Time: 15 Minutes.

Servings: 4.

INGREDIENTS:

- 4 salmon fillets, boneless.
- 2 tablespoons avocado oil.
- A pinch of salt and black pepper.
- 1 tablespoon lime juice.
- 2 shallots, chopped.
- 2 tablespoons walnuts, chopped.
- 2 tablespoons parsley, chopped.

DIRECTIONS:

1. Heat up a pan with the oil over medium-high heat, add the shallots, stir and sauté for 2 minutes.

2. Add the fish and the other ingredients, cook for 6 minutes on each side, divide between plates and serve.

NUTRITION:

- Calories 276.
- Fat 14.2 g.
- Fiber 0.7 g.
- Carbs: 2.7 g.
- Protein: 35.8 g.

- **Chives Trout**

Preparation Time: 10 Minutes.

Cooking Time: 15 Minutes.

Servings: 5.

INGREDIENTS:

- 4 trout fillets, boneless.

- 2 shallots, chopped.

- A pinch of salt and black pepper.

- 3 tablespoons chives, chopped.

- 2 tablespoons avocado oil.

- 2 teaspoons lime juice.

DIRECTIONS:

1. Heat up a pan with the oil over medium heat, add the shallots and sauté them for 2 minutes.

2. Add the fish and the rest of the ingredients, cook for 5 minutes on each side, divide into plates, and serve.

NUTRITION:

- Calories: 320.

- Fat 12 g.

- Fiber 1 g.

- Carbs: 2 g.

- Protein: 24 g.

- **Salmon and Tomatoes**

Preparation Time: 10 Minutes.

Cooking Time: 25 Minutes.

Servings: 4.

INGREDIENTS:

- 2 tablespoons avocado oil.

- 4 salmon fillets, boneless.

- 1 cup cherry tomatoes, halved.

- 2 spring onions, chopped.

- ½ cup chicken stock.

- A pinch of salt and black pepper.

- ½ teaspoon rosemary, dried.

DIRECTIONS:

1. In a roasting pan, combine the fish with the oil and the other ingredients, introduce in the oven at 400°F and bake for 25 minutes.

2. Divide between plates and serve.

NUTRITION:

- Calories 200.

- Fat 12 g.

- Fiber 0 g.

- Carbs: 3 g.

- Protein: 21 g.

- **Trout and Mustard Sauce**

Preparation Time: 5 Minutes.

Cooking Time: 20 Minutes.

Servings: 5.

INGREDIENTS:

- 2 tablespoons olive oil.
- 2 garlic cloves, minced.
- 2 spring onions.
- 4 trout fillets, boneless.
- A pinch of salt and black pepper.
- Juice and zest of 1 lime.
- ½ cup heavy cream.
- 2 tablespoons chives.

DIRECTIONS:

1. Heat up a pan with the oil over medium heat, add the garlic and the spring onions, stir and sauté for 3 minutes.

2. Add the fish and cook it for 4 minutes on each side.

NUTRITION:

- Calories: 171.
- Fat: 5 g.
- Fiber: 1 g.
- Carbs: 6 g.
- Protein: 23 g.

- **Sea Bass and Olives**

Preparation Time: 10 Minutes.

Cooking Time: 20 Minutes.

Servings: 5.

INGREDIENTS:

- 4 sea bass fillets, boneless.
- 2 tablespoons avocado oil.
- A pinch of salt and black pepper.
- 1 cup kalamata olives, pitted and sliced.
- 1 tablespoon oregano.
- 2 tablespoons capers.
- 1 tablespoon lime juice.
- 1 tablespoon cilantro.

DIRECTIONS:

1. Heat up a pan with the oil over medium heat, add the fish and cook it for 4 minutes on each side.

2. Add the olives and the other ingredients, toss gently, cook over medium-low heat for 10 minutes more, divide into plates and serve.

NUTRITION:

- Calories: 245
- Fat: 12 g.
- Fiber: 1 g.
- Carbs: 3 g.
- Protein: 23 g.

- **Paprika Shrimp Mix**

Preparation Time: 10 Minutes.

Cooking Time: 10 Minutes.

Servings: 5.

INGREDIENTS:

- 1 pound shrimp, peeled and deveined
- 3 garlic cloves, minced.
- 2 shallots, minced.
- 2 tablespoons olive oil.
- Juice of 1 lime.
- 2 teaspoons sweet paprika.
- 2 tablespoons parsley, chopped.

DIRECTIONS:

1. Heat up a pan with the oil over medium heat, add the garlic and the shallots, stir and cook for 2 minutes.

2. Add the shrimp and the other ingredients, cook over medium heat for 8 minutes more, divide between plates and serve.

NUTRITION:

- Calories: 205.
- Fat: 9.1 g.
- Fiber: 0.6 g.
- Carbs: 4.1 g.
- Protein: 26.2 g.

3. In the meantime, mash and add some lemon with your avocado.

4. Put it all together now, and season with salt and pepper. Perfect.

NUTRITION:

- Calories: 194.

- Fat: 4 g.

- Carbs: 26 g.

- Protein: 6 g.

- Sodium: 283 g.

LEGUMES AND VEGETABLES

- **Tomato Avocado Toast**

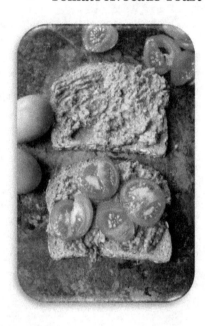

Preparation Time: 5 Minutes.

Cooking Time: 5 Minutes.

Servings: 5.

INGREDIENTS:

- 1 slice bread (ideally whole grain).

- ½ medium avocado (½ avocado = about 50g).

- 1 tbsp. lemon juice.

- 1 tbsp. olive oil.

- Salt and pepper to taste.

- Cherry tomatoes.

DIRECTIONS:

1. Split in half your cherry tomatoes.

2. Dump them in a pan and let them cook until tender (about 5 minutes) with olive oil.

- **Avocado Toast with Cottage Cheese**

Preparation Time: 5 minutes.

Cooking Time: 0 minutes.

Serves: 1.

INGREDIENTS:

- 1 green onion
- 2 tbsp. cottage cheese
- 1 tbsp. lemon
- ½ medium avocado
- 1 slice bread (ideally whole grain)
- salt and pepper to taste

DIRECTIONS:

1. Mash the avocado; add the lemon and some salt.
2. On the toast, put a layer of cottage cheese.
3. Garnish with fresh pepper and sliced green onion. Awe-inspirational!

NUTRITION:

- Calories: 194.
- Fat: 4 g.
- Carbs: 26 g.
- Protein: 6 g.
- Sodium: 283 g.

- **Creamy Corn Soup**

Preparation Time: 5 minutes.

Cooking Time: 15 minutes.

Servings: 4.

INGREDIENTS:

- 1 pinch pepper (preferably freshly ground black pepper)
- 1 pinch salt
- 2 handfuls cilantro/coriander, fresh
- 2 tbsp. olive oil
- 2 cups vegetable broth (2 cups = ½ liter)
- 1 thumb ginger, fresh (or 1 tbsp. ground ginger)
- 2 cloves garlic
- 1 red pepper
- 2 onions
- Cans sweet corn (ca. 14oz. or 350-400g cans)
- Optional and highly recommended:
- 1 tbsp. lemon juice (as an extra twist before serving)
- 2 stalks lemongrass (or 1 tbsp. ground lemongrass)

DIRECTIONS:

1. Heat the oven to a temperature of 430°F/220°C.
2. Flush the sweet corn in a different bowl, but save the water from the can!
3. To the baking tray, add ⅓ of the corn (without the water). Sprinkle with some salt, pepper, and oil. Put it on for about 10 minutes in the oven. Stir periodically to make sure the maize is not burning.
4. Meanwhile, heat the remaining tablespoon of oil in a pan over medium heat.
5. Chop and sauté the onion (slowly fry it).
6. Peel the fresh ginger and chop it and transfer it to the onion. (Keep off a moment if dried ginger is used). For a moment, stir.
7. The garlic is sliced and added to the onion. Stir for around 30–60 seconds when the heat is low.
8. Now's the time to apply that to the mix and swirl for around 30–60 seconds if you're using freshly grated ginger (and optional: ground lemongrass).
9. Put the other 2 cans of corn and the liquid you set aside earlier (with the water moist broth from the can). The vegetable broth is also added and brought to a boil.
10. Make tiny slits in the lemongrass and apply them to the soup if you're using fresh lemongrass. Or, to slap the lemongrass a few times, use a wooden spoon. Later, as a whole, you can pull them out, so make sure that they remain in one piece.
11. Let the soup boil on medium heat for around 10 minutes.
12. Regularly check on your oven-roasted corn. Meanwhile, cut the cilantro and slice the red pepper into small bits. If you don't want it hot, you want the red pepper first.
13. When the roasted corn is done (superbly golden, piping hot, popping here and there), put in the red pepper and coriander together to a cup. Just blend it well.

14. Remove the soup from the heat after ten minutes of boiling and mix it (a hand blender is ideal) until it's (kind of) smooth.

15. Serve the soup with the corn-coriander-red pepper mix in a teaspoon (or two!) of it.

NUTRITION:

- Calories: 194.

- Fat: 4 g.

- Carbs: 26 g.

- Protein: 6 g.

- Sodium: 283 g.

- **Egg on Avocado Toast**

Preparation Time: 5 minutes.

Cooking Time: 3 minutes.

Servings: 1.

INGREDIENTS:

- Slice bread.

- Salt and pepper to taste.

- 1 tbsp. olive oil.

- Sriracha.

- 1 egg.

- 1 tbsp. lemon.

- ½ medium avocado.

DIRECTIONS:

1. On medium-high heat, fry the egg and the toast in the pan with the olive oil.

2. In the meantime, mash the avocado, add salt and pepper, and put some lemon to the mixture.

3. Now add an egg to your toast.

4. Put a little bit of Sriracha and munches (or your favorite spicy sauce).

NUTRITION:

- Calories: 194.

- Fat: 4 g.

- Carbs: 26 g.

- Protein: 6 g.

- Sodium: 283 g.

- **Buckwheat Noodles with Veggies**

Preparation Time: 20 minutes.

Cooking Time: 25 minutes.

Servings: 2.

INGREDIENTS:

- 8 ounces buckwheat noodles.
- 2 tablespoons olive oil.
- 1 shallot, minced.
- 1 cup fresh mushrooms, sliced.
- 2 carrots, peeled and sliced diagonally.
- 1½ cup bok choy, chopped.
- 1/3 cup low-sodium vegetable broth.
- 1 tablespoon low-sodium soy sauce.

DIRECTIONS:

1. Bring lightly salted water in a pan to boil, cook the soba noodles for about 5 minutes.
2. Drain the noodles well and rinse under cold water. Set aside.
3. Over medium heat, heat the oil in a large wok and sauté the shallots for about 3 minutes.
4. Add the mushrooms and stir fry for about 4−5 minutes.
5. Add carrots and fry for 3 minutes while stirring.
6. Add bok choy and stir fry for about 2−3 minutes.
7. Add broth and simmer for about 2 minutes.
8. Add soy sauce and noodles and cook for about 1−2 minutes, tossing occasionally.
9. Serve hot.

NUTRITION:

- Calories: 224.
- Fat: 1 g.
- Carbs: 2 g.
- Protein: 6 g.
- Sodium: 398 g.

- **Eggplant Curry**

Preparation Time: 5 minutes.

Cooking Time: 30 minutes.

Servings: 2.

INGREDIENTS:

- ½ tbsp. pepper.
- ½ cups coconut milk (1 cup = 250ml).
- tin tomatoes (chopped) (roughly 14oz./400g).
- tbsp. ground coriander.
- tbsp. turmeric.
- 1 tbsp. gram masala powder or curry powder.
- clove garlic.
- 1 red onion.
- tbsp. olive oil.
- ½ tbsp. salt.
- 1 aborigine (medium).
- Optional:
- tbsp. sugar (or 1-2 tbsp. mango chutney).

DIRECTIONS

1. Cook as per packet directions when using rice.
2. Break your aubergine into tiny cubes. Fry with olive oil in a wide pan over high heat for 3–4 minutes. Mix well enough that it won't smoke.
3. Meanwhile, chop the onion, and put it in as well. Put it back to medium heat and cook for 5–6 minutes.
4. Crush the garlic or dice it.

5. Garlic, curry powder, turmeric, and ground cilantro should be mixed in. Cook, stirring well, for the next 3–4 minutes.
6. Add in the sliced tomatoes and coconut milk. Add salt.
7. Boil for 15 minutes, roughly.
8. The coconut milk gets thicker, so when it is at the right consistency for you, stop cooking.
9. If you like it a little sweeter, stir in the honey or mango chutney.
10. Serve with salt and pepper according to taste.

NUTRITION:

- Calories: 194.
- Fat: 4 g.
- Carbs: 26 g.
- Protein: 6 g.
- Sodium: 283 g.

- **Sweet Potato Soup**

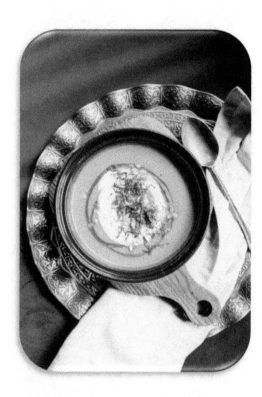

Preparation Time: 10 minutes.

Cooking Time: 20 minutes.

Servings: 4.

INGREDIENTS:

- 2 tbsp. olive oil.
- medium onion.
- 1 Bell pepper, red (yellow or red go well, but any will do).
- Cloves garlic (2 cloves = 1 tbsp. dried garlic).
- ½tbsp. cinnamon.
- 0.7 inches ginger, fresh (0.7 inches = 2 cm = 1 tbsp. dried ginger).
- 2 cups vegetable broth.
- 1 tbsp. peanut butter.
- ½ tbsp. cayenne pepper.
- ½ cup tomato puree.
- large sweet potato (approx. 300 g/ 10 oz. each; a total of 2.5 cups chopped).
- tbsp. soy sauce (low sodium if necessary).
- salt and pepper to taste.
- ½2½tbsp. vinegar (lemon juice can also be used).
- 2 tbsp. maple syrup.
- ½peanuts (to garnish).
- ½ lime (juiced).
- ¼ cup cilantro/coriander, fresh (Or other fresh herbs: go a bit wild with them—make it your signature dish by throwing in any and all of the following herbs that you have: basil, parsley, coriander, oregano).

DIRECTIONS:

1. Cut the onions and dump them into the oil in a pot on low to moderate heat. For around five minutes, let the onion cook steadily; it should begin to turn transparent.

2. Peel and then slice the sweet potatoes into chunks.

3. Cut the garlic, bell pepper, and ginger and put them into the bowl. Add them now if you're using dried herbs. Also, put in cinnamon and cayenne pepper. Cook and add the soy sauce, peanut butter, vinegar, and tomato for the next two minutes.

4. Stir well and apply a shot of broth.

5. Chuck in the sweet potatoes and most of the broth, and boil on medium heat. Add them now if you are using raw herbs. Stir regularly and after 10–15 minutes, confirm

the sweet potatoes are cooked (poke one with a knife and it should slip in).

6. Season using salt and pepper, maple syrup and lime juice and allow another swirl. If you used a cinnamon stick, then throw it out now.

7. Use a hand liquidizer or offer the soup a blend (blender if you do not have one). This is it—done!

8. Garnish with peanuts and serve with a side if desired—fresh bread is an obvious option!

NUTRITION

- Calories: 224.

- Fat: 1 g.

- Carbs: 2 g.

- Protein: 6 g.

- Sodium: 398 g.

- **Roasted Garlic Wilted Spinach**

Preparation Time: 5 minutes.

Cooking Time: 30 minutes.

Servings: 4.

INGREDIENTS:

- 1 tablespoon Garlic and Spring Onion Seasoning.
- 12 cup Baby spinach, rinsed.
- 2 tablespoon Roasted Garlic Oil.

DIRECTIONS:

1. Heat oil over high heat in an 8-quart pot until sizzling.
2. Apply the spinach and the seasoning and brush with a toss.
3. Put a lid on the pot and switch off the heat.
4. Leave it for about 3 minutes to allow it to set.
5. Take off the cover and throw the spinach once more. It's meant to be light green and actually wilted.

NUTRITION:

- Calories: 194.
- Fat: 4.
- Carbs: 26.
- Protein: 6.
- Sodium: 283.

- **Avocado Hummus**

Preparation Time: 10 minutes

Cooking Time: 0 minutes.

Servings: 6.

INGREDIENTS:

- ½ can chickpeas.
- ½tbsp. paprika powder.
- 1 tbsp. olive oil.
- ½ tbsp. pepper.
- ½ tbsp. salt.
- ½ tbsp. cumin.
- 1 cloves garlic.
- ½ lemon (juiced; lime works too).
- Medium ripe avocado.

DIRECTIONS

1. Drain the chickpeas and make sure to conserve water.
2. Peel and deseed your avocados-remember to clean off the dark green bits next to the skin! This is the healthiest part.
3. Juice the lemon and peel then finely cut the garlic.
4. Bringing all the items together into a food mixer.
5. Add ¼ cup chickpea water and mix for around a minute (you may also use plain water).
6. Put it all to a serving bowl and add the paprika powder on top to give it a good colorful finish.
7. Finished, that's it. Quick!
8. Time to enjoy your awesome dip.

NUTRITION

- Calories: 194.
- Fat: 4 g.
- Carbs: 26 g.
- Protein: 6 g.
- Sodium: 283 g.

- **Indian Lentil Soup**

Preparation Time: 10 minutes.

Cooking Time: 50 minutes.

Servings: 2.

INGREDIENTS:

- 2 cups of lentils.
- 1 small red onion, minced.
- 1 stalk of celery, finely chopped.
- 1 carrot, chopped.
- 2 large leaves of kale, chopped finely.
- 2 sprigs of cilantro, minced.
- 3 sprigs of parsley, minced.
- ¼–½ chili pepper, deseeded and minced.
- 1 tomato, chopped into small pieces.
- 1 chunk of ginger, minced.
- 1 clove of garlic, minced.
- 5 cups of chicken or vegetable stock.
- 1 tsp. of turmeric.
- 1 tsp. extra virgin olive oil.
- ½ tsp. Salt.

DIRECTIONS:

1. Cook lentils according to the package, removing from heat about 5 minutes before they would be done.
2. In a saucepan, sauté all of the vegetables in the olive oil.
3. Then add the chopped greens last.
4. Then add the ginger, garlic, and chill, and turmeric powder.
5. Add the stock and simmer for 5 minutes.
6. Add the lentils and salt.
7. Stir in the pre-cooked lentils and cook longer, on a very low simmer, for 25 more minutes.
8. Remove from the heat and cool.
9. Cut the avocado, remove the pit, and slice it, then scoop out the slices just before eating.
10. Top with avocado slice, then serve immediately.

NUTRITION:

- Calories 194.
- Fat: 4 g.
- Carbs 26 g.
- Protein 6 g.
- Sodium 283 g.

- **Green Beans**

Preparation Time: 5 minutes.

Cooking Time: 13 minutes.

Servings: 4.

INGREDIENTS:

- 1 pound green beans.
- ¾ teaspoon garlic powder.
- ¾ teaspoon ground black pepper.
- 1 ¼ teaspoon salt.
- ½ teaspoon paprika.

DIRECTIONS:

1. Meanwhile, place beans in a bowl, spray generously with olive oil, sprinkle with garlic powder, black pepper, salt, and paprika and toss until well coated.

2. Open the fryer, add green beans to it, close with its lid and cook for 8 minutes until nicely golden and crispy, shaking halfway through the frying.

3. When the air fryer beeps, open its lid, transfer green beans onto a serving plate and serve.

NUTRITION:

- Calories: 45.
- Carbs: 2 g.
- Fat: 11 g.
- Protein: 4 g.
- Fiber: 3 g.

- **Asparagus Avocado Soup**

Preparation Time: 10 minutes.

Cooking Time: 20 minutes.

Servings: 4.

INGREDIENTS:

- 1 avocado, peeled, pitted, cubed.
- 12 ounces asparagus.
- ½ teaspoon ground black pepper.
- 1 teaspoon garlic powder.
- 1 teaspoon sea salt.
- 2 tablespoons olive oil, divided.
- 1/2 of a lemon, juiced.
- 2 cups vegetable stock.

DIRECTIONS:

1. Meanwhile, place asparagus in a shallow dish, drizzle with 1-tablespoon oil, sprinkle with garlic powder, salt, and black pepper, and toss until well mixed.

2. Open the fryer, add asparagus to it, close with its lid and cook for 10 minutes until nicely golden and roasted, shaking halfway through the frying.

3. When the air fryer beeps, open its lid and transfer asparagus to a food processor.

4. Add remaining ingredients into a food processor and pulse until well combined and smooth.

5. Tip the soup in a saucepan, pour in water if the soup is too thick, and heat it over medium-low heat for 5 minutes until thoroughly heated.

6. Ladle soup into bowls and serve.

NUTRITION:

- Calories: 208.
- Carbs: 2 g.
- Fat: 11 g.
- Protein: 4 g.
- Fiber: 5 g.

- **Sweet Potato Chips**

Preparation Time: 5 minutes.

Cooking Time: 10 minutes.

Servings: 4.

INGREDIENTS:

- 2 large sweet potatoes.

- 15 ml. of oil.

- 10 g of salt.

- 2 g black pepper.

- 2 g of paprika.

- 2 g garlic powder.

- 2 g onion powder.

DIRECTIONS:

1. Cut the sweet potatoes into strips 25 mm thick.

2. Preheat the air fryer for a few minutes.

3. Add the cut sweet potatoes to a large bowl and mix with the oil until the potatoes are all evenly coated.

4. Sprinkle salt, black pepper, paprika, garlic powder, and onion powder. Mix well.

5. Place the French fries in the preheated baskets and cook for 10 minutes at 205°C (400°F). Be sure to shake the baskets halfway through cooking.

NUTRITION:

- Calories: 123.

- Carbs: 2 g.

- Fat: 11 g.

- Protein: 4 g.

- Fiber: 0 g.

- **Fried Zucchini**

Preparation Time: 10 minutes.

Cooking Time: 8 minutes.

Servings: 4.

INGREDIENTS:

- 2 medium zucchinis.
- 60g all-purpose flour.
- 12g of salt.
- 2g black pepper.
- 2 beaten eggs.
- 15 ml of milk.
- 84g Italian seasoned breadcrumbs.
- 25g grated Parmesan cheese.
- Non-stick Spray Oil.
- Ranch sauce, to serve.

DIRECTIONS:

1. Cut the zucchini into strips 19 mm thick.
2. Mix with the flour, salt, and pepper on a plate. Mix the eggs and milk in a separate dish.
3. Cover each piece of zucchini with flour, then dip them in egg and pass them through the crumbs. Leave aside.
4. Preheat the air fryer, set it to 175°C (345°F).
5. Place the covered zucchini in the preheated air fryer and spray with oil spray. Set the timer to 8 minutes and press Start/Pause.
6. Be sure to shake the baskets in the middle of cooking.
7. Serve with tomato sauce or ranch sauce.

NUTRITION:

- Calories: 68.
- Carbs: 2 g.
- Fat: 11 g.
- Protein: 4 g.
- Fiber: 143 g.

- **Fried Avocado**

Preparation Time: 15 minutes.

Cooking Time: 10 minutes.

Servings: 2.

INGREDIENTS:

- 2 avocados.
- 50g Pan crumbs bread.
- 2g garlic powder.
- 2g onion powder.
- 1g smoked paprika.
- 1g cayenne pepper.
- Salt and pepper to taste.
- 60g all-purpose flour.
- 2 eggs, beaten.
- Non-stick Spray Oil.
- Tomato sauce or ranch sauce, to serve.

DIRECTIONS:

1. Cut the avocados into 25 mm thick pieces.
2. Combine the crumbs, garlic powder, onion powder, smoked paprika, cayenne pepper, and salt in a bowl.
3. Separate each wedge of avocado in the flour, then dip the beaten eggs and stir in the breadcrumb mixture.
4. Preheat the air fryer.
5. Turn the fried avocado halfway through cooking and sprinkle with cooking oil.
6. Serve with tomato sauce or ranch sauce.

NUTRITION:

- Calories: 123.
- Carbs: 2 g.
- Fat: 11 g.
- Protein: 4 g.
- Fiber: 0 g.

- **Vegetables in Air Fryer**

Preparation time: 20 minutes

Cooking time: 30 minutes

Servings: 2

INGREDIENTS:

- 2 potatoes.

- 1 zucchini.

- 1 onion.

- 1 red pepper.

- 1 green pepper.

DIRECTIONS:

1. Cut the potatoes into slices.

2. Cut the onion into rings.

3. Cut the zucchini slices

4. Cut the peppers into strips.

5. Put all the ingredients in the bowl and add a little salt, ground pepper, and some extra virgin olive oil.

6. Mix well.

7. Pass to the basket of the air fryer.

8. Select 160°C (320°F), 30 minutes.

9. Check that the vegetables are to your liking.

NUTRITION:

- Calories: 135.

- Carbs: 2 g.

- Fat: 11 g.

- Protein: 4 g.

- Fiber: 05 g.

- **Crispy Rye Bread Snacks with Guacamole and Anchovies**

Preparation Time: 10 minutes.

Cooking Time: 10 minutes.

Servings: 4.

INGREDIENTS:

- 4 slices of rye bread.

- Guacamole.

- Anchovies in oil.

DIRECTIONS:

1. Cut each slice of bread into 3 strips of bread.

2. Place in the basket of the air fryer, without piling up, and we go in batches giving it the touch you want to give it. You can select 180°C (350°F), 10 minutes.

3. When you have all the crusty rye bread strips, put a layer of guacamole on top, whether homemade or commercial.

4. In each bread, place 2 anchovies on the guacamole.

NUTRITION:

- Calories: 180

- Carbs: 4 g

- Fat: 11 g

- Protein: 4 g

- Fiber: 09 g

- **Beef with Grilled Vegetables**

Preparation Time: 10 minutes.

Cooking Time: 30 minutes.

Servings: 1.

INGREDIENTS:

- 4 sirloin steaks
- 2 tbsp. olive oil
- 3 tbsp. balsamic vinegar

Vegetables:

- ½ lb. asparagus, trimmed
- 1 cup green beans
- 1 cup snow peas
- 1 red bell peppers, cut into strips
- 1 orange bell peppers, cut into strips
- 1 medium red onion, quartered

DIRECTIONS:

1. Set a grill pan over high heat.
2. Grab 2 separate bowls and put the beef in one and the vegetables in another.
3. Mix salt, pepper, olive oil, and balsamic vinegar in a small bowl and pour half of the mixture over the beef and the other half over the vegetables.
4. Coat the ingredients in both bowls with the sauce.
5. Place the steaks in the grill pan and sear both sides for 2–3 minutes each.
6. When done, remove the beef onto a plate; set aside.
7. Pour the vegetables and marinade in the pan and cook for 5 minutes, turning once.
8. Share the vegetables on plates.
9. Top with beef, drizzle the sauce from the pan all over and serve.

NUTRITION:

- Calories: 194.
- Fat: 4.
- Carbs: 26.
- Protein: 6.
- Sodium: 283.

SWEET TOOTH SNACKS & DESSERT

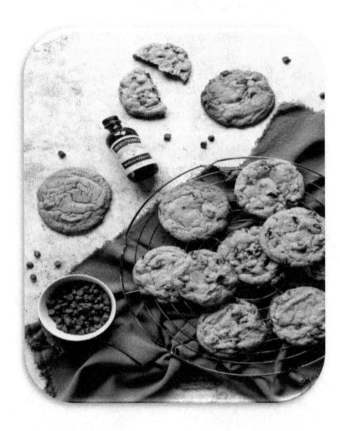

- **Triple Chocolate Chip Deep Dish Cookies**

Preparation Time: 10 minutes.

Cooking Time: 30 minutes.

Servings: 1.

INGREDIENTS:

- 3/4 cup canned pumpkin.
- 3/4 cup chocolate peanut butter.
- 1/2 cup powdered chocolate protein.
- 1/4 cup honey.
- 1 beaten egg.
- 1 teaspoon pure vanilla.
- 1/2 teaspoon baking soda.
- 1/2 cup sugar-free chocolate chips.
- Vanilla ice cream or serving.

DIRECTIONS:

1. Add all the ingredients except ice cream and chocolate chips to a bowl
2. Use a mixer (electric) beat until mixed evenly.
3. Heat your oven to 350°F.
4. Gradually add the chocolate chips and gently fold to incorporate.
5. Pour batter into a skillet (medium).
6. Place skillet into a preheated oven to bake for approximately 20 minutes until golden brown.
7. Remove from heat and set aside for roughly 7–10 minutes.
8. Serve using the vanilla ice cream.

NUTRITION:

- Calories: 502.
- Protein: 6 g.
- Carbohydrates: 65 g.
- Fats: 24 g.

- **Protein Brownies**

Preparation Time: 10 minutes.

Cooking Time: 30–35 minutes.

Servings: 1.

INGREDIENTS:

- 1/2 cup almond milk.

- 1/2 cup chocolate flavored egg whites.

- 1/2 cup unsweetened apple sauce.

- 1/2 cup + 1 tablespoon Greek yogurt.

- 1 cup oat flour.

- 2–3 scoops, powdered chocolate protein.

- 3 tablespoon powdered unsweetened cocoa.

- 1 teaspoon baker style baking powder.

- 1/2 teaspoon salt.

Frosting:

- 1/2 cup non-fat Greek yogurt.

- 1/4 cup cherries.

- Sweetener (optional).

DIRECTIONS:

1. The first step is to heat an oven to 350°F, then lightly spray a baking dish using cooking spray.

2. Add the egg whites and whisk well until beaten lightly.

3. Add the protein powder, oat flour, sweetener, powdered cocoa, and baking powder separately.

4. Stir well until mixed evenly, then pour milk mixture (almond) into the flour mixture.

5. Stir well until thoroughly mixed and set batter aside for approximately 5 minutes.

6. Pour batter into the dish and place into the oven to bake for approximately 25 minutes until thoroughly cooked.

7. Remove brownie from heat, then set aside to cool.

8. Add all the frosting ingredients in a food processor, then process on the highest setting until it becomes smooth.

9. Spread frosting over the top of brownies. Serve.

NUTRITION:

- Calories: 466.

- Protein: 6 g.

- Carbohydrates: 50 g.

- Fats: 29 g.

- **Protein Pumpkin Spiced Donuts**

Preparation Time: 10 minutes.

Cooking Time: 15 minutes.

Servings: 1.

INGREDIENTS:

- 1 cup oat flour.
- 3/4 cup xylitol.
- 1 scoop powdered vanilla protein.
- 1 tablespoon ground flaxseed.
- 1 tablespoon ground cinnamon.
- 2 teaspoons baking powder.
- 1 teaspoon sea salt.
- 3 beaten eggs.
- 1/2 cup canned pumpkin.
- 1 tablespoon melted coconut oil.
- 2 teaspoons pure vanilla.
- 1 teaspoon apple cider vinegar.

Frosting:

- 1/2 cup whipped cream cheese
- 1/2 teaspoon liquid stevia.

DIRECTIONS:

1. Place the xylitol, oat flour, ground flaxseed, powdered protein, baking powder, ground cinnamon, and a dash of sea salt in a large bowl. Preheat your oven to 350°F.

2. Add the egg (beaten) into another bowl (large) along with the pumpkin (canned), pure vanilla, and vinegar, and coconut oil (melted).

3. Whisk until mixed (evenly), then pour the mixture into the flour. Stir until thoroughly mixed.

4. Use cooking spray grease a large donut pan.

5. Pour batter into the donut pan (greased).

6. Place batter into the oven and bake for approximately 10 minutes until thoroughly baked.

7. Remove from heat and set donuts onto a wire rack to cool.

8. Add in the cream cheese (whipped) and liquid stevia in a small bowl, whisk until it becomes smooth.

9. Frost donuts using the frosting and serve with a sprinkle of cinnamon (ground) over the top.

NUTRITION:

- Calories: 452.
- Protein: 4.9 g.
- Carbohydrates: 51 g.
- Fats: 25 g.

- **High Protein Chipotle Cheddar Quesadilla**

Preparation Time: 15 Minutes.

Cooking Time: 45 Minutes.

Servings: 1.

INGREDIENTS:

- 1 low-carb tortillas.

- 1/2 cup low sodium cottage cheese.

- 1/2 cups low fat, shredded cheddar cheese.

- 1/4 red thinly sliced bell pepper.

- 1/4 thinly sliced onion.

- 1/4 cup thinly sliced portobello mushrooms.

- 1 tablespoon chipotle seasoning.

- Mild salsa (for dipping).

DIRECTIONS:

1. Add the bell pepper (sliced, red), onion (sliced), and mushrooms (sliced) into a large grill pan over medium heat.

2. Cook for approximately 10 minutes until soft. Remove then transfer into a bowl (medium). Set aside.

3. Add the chipotle seasoning and cottage cheese in a small bowl. Stir well to incorporate.

4. Place tortillas onto the grill pan and pour vegetable mixture over tortillas.

5. Sprinkle cottage cheese mixture over the top, then top off using the cheddar cheese (shredded).

6. Place an additional tortilla over the top of the filling.

7. Cook for roughly 2 minutes, then flip and continue cooking for the next minute.

8. Repeat process with remaining tortillas and filling. 9. Serve immediately with the salsa (mild).

NUTRITION:

- Calories: 293.

- Protein: 15 g.

- Carbohydrates: 24 g.

- Fats: 15 g.

- **Sweet Potato Casserole**

Preparation Time: 5 Minutes.

Cooking Time: 15 Minutes.

Servings: 1.

INGREDIENTS:

- 1/2 pounds sweet, peeled, and chopped potatoes

- 1/3 cup nonfat Greek yogurt.

- 1/2 tablespoon ground cinnamon.

- 1/8 teaspoon ground nutmeg.

- 1/4 teaspoon sea salt.

- 1 tablespoon egg whites.

- 1/4 tablespoon melted butter.

- 1/2 cup chopped pecans

- 1/2 cup miniature marshmallows

- Sugar (dash, light brown, for sprinkling)

DIRECTIONS:

1. Heat your oven to 375°F.

2. Place the potatoes (sweet) into a saucepan (large) over medium-high heat.

3. Cover potatoes using water, then bring to a boil, boil for approximately 30 minutes until soft.

4. Drain potatoes, then place potatoes back into the saucepan.

5. Add the Greek yogurt, cinnamon (ground), nutmeg (ground), and sea salt (dash) into the potatoes.

6. Stir well until coated (evenly).

7. Add in the butter (melted) and egg whites, then bring to a stir once more.

8. Transfer potato mixture into a casserole dish (large).

9. Place into the oven, then bakes for approximately 30 minutes. Remove from heat, then top with the pecans (chopped) and miniature marshmallows.

10. Place back into the oven to bake for an additional 10 minutes until marshmallows are browned.

NUTRITION:

- Calories: 86.

- Protein: 1.6 g.

- Carbohydrates: 20 g.

- Fats: 0.1 g.

- **Barbecue Pulled Pork Sandwiches**

- Fats: 10g.

Preparation Time: 10 Minutes.

Cooking Time: 6 hours.

Servings: 1.

INGREDIENTS:

- ¼ pound pork tenderloin.

- 1/4 cup barbecue sauce.

- 1 hamburger rolls.

- 1/2 cup shredded coleslaw.

- 1/2 cup Greek yogurt.

- 1 ½ tablespoon Dijon mustard.

- Salt and black pepper (dash).

DIRECTIONS:

1. Add in the pork tenderloin into a slow cooker, then pour barbecue sauce over the top.

2. Cover using the lid and cook for 6 hours on medium setting until soft.

3. Remove pork tenderloin and finely shred using two forks.

4. Add in the yogurt, coleslaw, and Dijon mustard into a small-sized bowl and season using a dash of salt and black pepper. Stir until thoroughly mixed.

5. Divide pork among hamburger buns, then tops off using the coleslaw.

6. Serve immediately.

NUTRITION:

- Calories: 155.

- Protein: 34g.

- Carbohydrates: 28g.

- **Sweet Cinnamon Rolls**

Preparation Time: 10 Minutes.

Cooking Time: 20 Minutes.

Servings: 1.

INGREDIENTS:

Dough:

- ¼ cup Oat flour extra for rolling.

- 1 tablespoon coconut sugar.

- 1 teaspoon baking powder.

- ½ teaspoon Xanthium gum.

- 1/2 tablespoon cold coconut oil.

- 1 to 2 tablespoons whole milk.

Filling:

- 1 tablespoon melted coconut oil.

- ½ tablespoon ground cinnamon.

- 2 tablespoons coconut sugar.

Frosting:

- ¼ cup Greek yogurt.

- 1 to 2 tablespoons whole milk.

- 1 tablespoon vanilla protein.

- Pecans.

DIRECTIONS:

1. Preheat the oven to 400°F.

2. In a bowl (large), put in all the ingredients for the dough. Stir thoroughly to mix until your dough becomes soft. Before putting it into the fridge, cover the dough and allow chill for about 20 minutes.

3. Put the dough onto a flat surface that has been dusted with flour. Roll the dough into a square (large).

4. Spread half of the coconut oil over the top part of the dough. Use coconut sugar and ground cinnamon to sprinkle over the top.

5. Using jelly-roll style, roll the dough. Slice the dough into rolls. Place onto a baking sheet (large) with the side that was cut facing down.

6. Spread the coconut oil over the top of the rolls.

7. Place cinnamon rolls into the oven to bake for approximately 20 minutes. 8. For 10 minutes, let it cool, then serve.

NUTRITION:

- Calories: 436.

- Protein: 4.7 g.

- Carbohydrates: 50 g.

- Fats: 24 g.

- **Puffed Brown Rice**

Preparation Time: 55 Minutes.

Cooking Time: 15 Minutes.

Servings: 1.

INGREDIENTS:

- 1/4 cup dry and brown rice.

- 1–2 cups MCT oil.

DIRECTIONS:

1. Use paper towels to line a medium bowl.

2. In a saucepan, pour 5–8 cups of MCT oil and heat over medium-high heat.

3. Ensure that saucepan is fully covered with oil.

4. Once the oil is hot enough, place the rice grains (dry) using a sieve until the pot is fully covered with rice.

5. Gently shake to ensure everything puffs up. Be careful not to burn the rice.

6. Remove sieve with the rice (puffed), then transfer puffed grains into the bowl.

7. Set aside to let cool, then discard the leftover oil.

8. Once cooled. Enjoy.

NUTRITION:

- Calories: 402.

- Protein: 6 g.

- Carbohydrates: 90 g.

- Fats: 0.5 g.

- **Homemade Chocolates with Coconut and Raisins**

- Protein: 1.3 g.

Preparation Time: 10 Minutes.

Cooking Time: 15 Minutes.

Servings: 5.

INGREDIENTS:

- 1/2 cup cacao butter, melted.

- 1/3 cup peanut butter.

- 1/4 cup agave syrup.

- A pinch of grated nutmeg.

- A bit of coarse salt.

- 1/2 teaspoon vanilla extract.

- 1 cup dried coconut, shredded.

- 6 oz. dark chocolate, chopped.

- 3 oz. raisins.

DIRECTIONS:

1. Carefully combine all the ingredients, not including the chocolate, in a mixing bowl.

2. Spoon the mixture into molds.

3. Leave to set hard in a cool place.

4. Melt the dark chocolate in your microwave.

5. Pour in the melted chocolate until the fillings are covered.

6. Leave to set hard in a cool place.

7. Enjoy!

NUTRITION:

- Calories: 130.

- Fat: 9.1 g.

- Carbs: 12.1 g.

- **Almond and Chocolate Chip Bars**

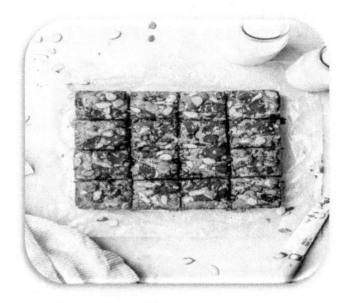

Preparation Time: 10 Minutes.

Cooking Time: 30 Minutes.

Servings: 1.

INGREDIENTS:

- 1/2 cup almond butter.
- 1/4 cup coconut oil, melted.
- 1/4 cup agave syrup.
- 1 teaspoon vanilla extract.
- 1/4 teaspoon sea salt.
- 1/4 teaspoon grated nutmeg.
- 1/2 teaspoon ground cinnamon.
- 2 cups almond flour.
- 1/4 cup flaxseed meal.
- 1 cup vegan chocolate, cut into chunks.
- 1 1/3 cups almonds, ground.
- 2 tablespoons cacao powder.
- 1/4 cup agave syrup.

DIRECTIONS:

- In a mixing bowl, thoroughly combine the almond butter, coconut oil, 1/4 cup of agave syrup, vanilla, salt, nutmeg, and cinnamon.
- Gradually stir in the almond flour and flaxseed meal and stir to combine. Add in the chocolate chunks and start again.
- In a small blending bowl, combine the almonds, cacao powder, and agave syrup. Now, spread the ganache onto the cake.
- Freeze for about 30 minutes, cut into bars, and serve well chilled.
- Enjoy!

NUTRITION:

- Calories: 295.
- Fat: 17 g.
- Carbs: 35.2 g.
- Protein: 1.7 g.

- **Easy Mocha Fudge**

Preparation Time: 10 Minutes.

Cooking Time: 60 Minutes.

Servings: 1.

INGREDIENTS:

- 1 cup cookies, crushed.

- 1/2 cup almond butter.

- 1/4 cup agave nectar.

- 6 oz. dark chocolate, broken into chunks.

- 1 teaspoon instant coffee.

- A pinch grated nutmeg.

- A pinch salt.

DIRECTIONS:

- Line a large baking layer with parchment paper.

- Melt the chocolate in your microwave and add in the remaining ingredients; stir to combine well.

- Scrape the batter into a parchment-lined baking sheet. Put it in your freezer for a minimum of 1 hour to set.

- Cut into squares and serve. Bon appétit!

NUTRITION:

- Calories: 105.

- Fat: 5.6 g.

- Carbs: 12.9 g.

- Protein: 1.1 g.

- **Wrapped Plums**

Preparation Time: 5 Minutes.

Cooking Time: 5 Minutes.

Servings: 5.

INGREDIENTS:

- 2 ounces prosciutto, cut into 16 pieces.

- 4 plums, quartered.

- 1 tablespoon chives, chopped.

- A pinch of red pepper flakes, crushed.

DIRECTIONS:

- Wrap each plum quarter in a prosciutto slice, and arrange them all on a platter.

- Sprinkle the chives and pepper flakes all over and serve.

NUTRITION:

- Calories: 30.

- Fat: 1 g.

- Fiber: 0 g.

- Carbs: 4 g.

- Protein: 2 g.

- **Cucumber Sandwich Bites**

Preparation Time: 5 Minutes.

Cooking Time: 0 Minutes.

Servings: 5.

INGREDIENTS:

- 1 cucumber, sliced.
- 8 slices whole-wheat bread.
- 2 tablespoons cream cheese, soft.
- 1 tablespoon chives, chopped.
- ¼ cup avocado, peeled, pitted, and mashed.
- 1 teaspoon mustard.
- Salt and black pepper to the taste.

DIRECTIONS:

- Spread the mashed avocado on each bread slice, also spread the rest of the ingredients except the cucumber slices.
- Divide the cucumber slices into the bread slices, cut each slice in thirds, arrange on a platter, and serve as an appetizer.

NUTRITION:

- Calories: 187.
- Fat: 12.4 g.
- Fiber: 2.1 g.
- Carbs: 4.5 g.
- Protein: 8.2 g.

- **Cucumber Rolls**

Preparation Time: 5 Minutes

Cooking Time: 0 Minutes

Servings: 5

INGREDIENTS:

- 1 big cucumber, sliced lengthwise.
- 1 tablespoon parsley, chopped.
- 8 ounces canned tuna, drained and mashed.
- Salt and black pepper to the taste.
- 1 teaspoon lime juice.

DIRECTIONS:

- Arrange cucumber slices on a working surface, divide the rest of the ingredients, and roll.
- Arrange all the rolls on a surface and serve as an appetizer.

NUTRITION:

- Calories: 200
- Fat: 6 g.
- Fiber: 3.4 g.
- Carbs: 7.6 g.
- Protein: 3.5 g.

- **Olives and Cheese Stuffed Tomatoes**

Preparation Time: 15 Minutes.

Cooking Time: 0 Minutes.

Servings: 20.

INGREDIENTS:

- 24 cherry tomatoes, top cut off, and insides scooped out.

- 2 tablespoons olive oil.

- ¼ teaspoon red pepper flakes.

- ½ cup feta cheese, crumbled.

- 2 tablespoons black olive paste.

- ¼ cup mint, torn.

DIRECTIONS:

- In a bowl, mix the olives paste with the rest of the ingredients except the cherry tomatoes and whisk well.

- Stuff the cherry tomatoes with this mix, arrange them all on a platter, and serve as an appetizer.

NUTRITION:

- Calories: 136.

- Fat: 8.6 g.

- Fiber: 4.8 g.

- Carbs: 5.6 g.

- Protein: 5.1 g.

- **Chocolate Bars**

Preparation Time: 5 Minutes.

Cooking Time: 25 Minutes.

Servings: 16.

INGREDIENTS:

- 15 oz. cream cheese, softened.
- 15 oz. unsweetened dark chocolate.
- 1 tsp. vanilla.
- 10 drops liquid stevia.

DIRECTIONS:

- Grease 8-inch square dish and set aside.
- In a saucepan, dissolve chocolate over low heat.
- Add stevia and vanilla and stir well.
- Remove pan from heat and set aside.
- Add cream cheese into the blender and blend until smooth.
- Add melted chocolate mixture into the cream cheese and blend until just combined.
- Transfer mixture into the prepared dish and spread evenly, and place in the refrigerator until firm.
- Slice and serve.

NUTRITION:

- Calories: 230.
- Fat: 24 g.
- Carbs: 7.5 g.
- Sugar: 0.1 g.
- Protein: 6 g.
- Cholesterol: 29 mg.

- **Blueberry Muffins**

Preparation Time: 15 Minutes.

Cooking Time: 45 Minutes.

Servings: 10.

INGREDIENTS:

- 2 eggs.

- 1/2 cup fresh blueberries.

- 1 cup heavy cream.

- 2 cups almond flour.

- 1/4 tsp. lemon zest.

- 1/2 tsp. lemon extract.

- 1 tsp. baking powder.

- 5 drops stevia.

- 1/4 cup butter, melted.

DIRECTIONS:

- Heat the cooker to 350°F.

- Line muffin tin with cupcake liners and set aside.

- Add eggs into the bowl and whisk until mix.

- Add remaining ingredients and mix to combine.

- Pour mixture into the prepared muffin tin and bake for 25 minutes.

- Serve and enjoy.

NUTRITION:

- Calories: 190.

- Fat: 17 g.

- Carbs: 5 g.

- Sugar: 1 g.

- Protein: 5 g.

- Cholesterol: 55 mg.

- **Chia Pudding**

Preparation Time: 5 Minutes.

Cooking Time: 15 Minutes.

Servings: 2.

INGREDIENTS:

- 4 tbsp. chia seeds.
- 1 cup unsweetened coconut milk.
- 1/2 cup raspberries.

DIRECTIONS:

- Add raspberry and coconut milk into a blender and blend until smooth.
- Pour mixture into the glass jar.
- Add chia seeds in a jar and stir well.
- Seal the jar with a lid and shake well and place in the refrigerator for 3 hours.
- Serve chilled and enjoy.

NUTRITION:

- Calories: 360.
- Fat: 33 g.
- Carbs: 13 g.
- Sugar: 5 g.
- Protein: 6 g.
- Cholesterol: 0 mg.

- **Avocado Pudding**

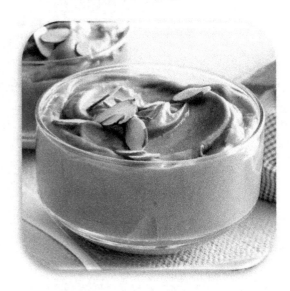

Preparation Time: 15 Minutes.

Cooking Time: 0 Minutes.

Servings: 5.

INGREDIENTS:

- 2 ripe avocados, pitted and cut into pieces.

- 1 tbsp. fresh lime juice.

- 14 oz. can coconut milk.

- 2 tsp. liquid stevia.

- 2 tsp. vanilla.

DIRECTIONS:

- Inside the blender, add all ingredients and blend until smooth.

- Serve immediately and enjoy.

NUTRITION:

- Calories: 317.

- Fat: 30 g.

- Carbs: 9 g.

- Sugar: 0.5 g.

- Protein: 3 g.

- Cholesterol: 0 mg.

CONCLUSION

T he Lean and Green diet is one of the most followed and effective diet programs.

Unlike other regimens, it is not designed for a specific health condition. It is designed according to the dietitian's needs to achieve the ideal weight and the healthy lifestyle you want.

The logic is that eating healthy recipes will make you feel full for a long time in contrast to foods that are high in carbohydrates and saturated fat. That's why it focuses on increasing the consumption of whole foods and reducing the use of fast commercial foods and other unhealthy foods.

The program has earned worldwide popularity for its ability to deliver sustainable results without complicating the meal program for people. It places very few restrictions on food and inspires people to choose a healthier version of their daily food without compromising on taste and nutrition.

Choosing the right diet or program had also become difficult as the industry flourished. Many diets claim to have specific health problems while helping a diet lose weight. The Lean and Green diet is the right solution!

CPSIA information can be obtained
at www.ICGtesting.com
Printed in the USA
BVHW061059010521
606211BV00011B/1620

9 781802 66